MW01181431

3 9049 00034 5100

your eyes!

A Comprehensive Look at the Understanding and Treatment of Vision Problems

Dr. Thomas L. D'Alonzo, O.D.

Avanti Publishing, Clifton Heights, Pennsylvania

YOUR EYES! A Comprehensive Look at the Understanding and
Treatment of Vision Problems

by T.L. D'Alonzo, O.D.

Published by: Avanti Publishing
P.O. Box 237
Clifton Heights, PA   19018   USA

© Copyright   1991 by Thomas L. D'Alonzo, O.D.
First printing 1991
Second printing 1992

Publisher's Cataloging in Publication (Prepared by Quality Books Inc.)

D'Alonzo, Thomas L., 1954-
   Your Eyes! : a comprehensive look at the understanding and
treatment of vision problems / Thomas L. D'Alonzo. –
   p. cm.
   Includes bibliographical references and index.
   ISBN 0-9629063-5-2
   1. Ophthalmology – Popular works.   2. Eye – Diseases and defects –
Popular works.   3. Eye-Care and hygiene – Popular works.   4. Vision
disorders – Popular works.   I. Title.

RE51   617.7
                                            QBI91-423
Library of Congress Catalog Card Number: 91-71193

All rights reserved. No part of this book may be reproduced or transmitted
in any form or by any other means, without written permission of the author,
except for the inclusion of brief quotations in a review.

Printed in the United States of America

FOREWORD

YOUR EYES! is written for everyone concerned about the health and care of their eyes. It attempts to address basic eye health and vision needs in a straightforward, non-technical manner. Many pictures and diagrams are used throughout the book to aid in the understanding of the concepts and descriptions. This book is designed for both easy reading and use as a reference.

Chapter One addresses the different types of eyecare practitioners, what an eye exam includes and symptoms of eye disorders.

The second and third chapters (anatomy and physiology) explain how the human eye functions. In order to understand function, a certain knowledge of anatomy is required. The pysiology chapter addresses the process of vision itself. This chapter also includes basic optics, color vision and the interrelationship between the eyes and the brain.

The chapter on refractive errors and their correction include basic descriptions of nearsightedness, farsightedness, astigmatism and presbyopia. The correction of these disorders with eyeglasses and contact lenses is considered in detail.

Visual disorders in children are found in Chapter Five: Visual Disorders Affecting Children and Young Adults. The complexities of childhood eye problems and their treatment are covered. Pediatric eye care problems include focusing difficulties, binocular vision problems, eyeturns and perceptual dysfunctions. Attention is also given to the normal development of the child. Treatment for these conditions emphasizes vision therapy which is covered in great length.

Sports vision and environmental eye care is addressed next. This chapter emphasizes eye safety and improved athletic performance through vision therapy and training exercises. The sports vision section covers the vision skills needed for sports and how these skills can be enhanced.

The next three chapters cover eye disease, medications and eye surgery. The chapters on eye disease and medications are covered from two approaches; eye disease and eye medications and also how systemic disorders and systemic medications can affect the eyes. Contact lens solutionsare also covered in the chapter on eye medications. The chapter on surgery stresses the description and prognosis of the most common eye surgery. Special attention is given to cataract surgery.

147400

Chapter Ten deals with the normal aging changes of the eye as well as sub-normal vision. Rehabilitation of the visually impaired, primarily with low vision aids, is covered in depth. The final chapter stresses prevention as a means of maintaining eye health and avoiding serious vision problems.

I hope **YOUR EYES!** helps answer most questions on eye care and eye health many people have. Individuals are taking a greater interest in their eyes, following the trend of increased interest in overall health and well being.

The purpose of **YOUR EYES!** is to stimulate interest in eye care and provide information in a straightforward yet, hopefully, enjoyable manner.

– Thomas L. D'Alonzo, O.D.

Contents

YOUR EYES!

WARNING DISCLAIMER

This book is designed to provide information in regard to the subject matter covered.

The purpose of this book is to educate and entertain.

It is sold with the understanding that the publisher and author shall have neither liability nor responsibility to any person with respect to any loss or damage caused or alleged to be caused directly or indirectly by the information contained in this book.

DEDICATION

This book is dedicated to my wife, Lisa and
my daughter, Angela.

I wish to thank Ed Petersen, commercial artist,
for his help on the illustrations and
SSS Electronic Publishing, Inc. for their help in
getting "**YOUR EYES!**" into print.

1

Introduction

The Eyecare Team

There are three major participants in eyecare: the ophthalmologist, the optometrist and the optician.

The American Optometric Association defines an optometrist as follows: the doctor of optometry is a primary health care provider who diagnoses, manages and treats conditions and diseases of the human eye and visual system as regulated by state law.

The optometrist is the major provider of primary eyecare in America today. Optometric education and clinical training is specific for eye disorders and their management. Optometric services, generally, include the following: a comprehensive examination of the inside and outside parts of the eye, an evaluation of the patient's vision, and diagnosis and treatment of the disorder.

The examination can detect eye diseases such as glaucoma and cataracts as well as systemic disorders including diabetes and hypertension. Diabetes and hypertension are frequently first detected during a comprehensive eye examination.

YOUR EYES!

The optometrist can perform a variety of tests to determine the patient's visual acuity, focusing ability, eye coordination and field of vision. Color vision and depth perception are also tested. An analysis of the information is made and the doctor arrives at a diagnosis.

Treatment may consist of prescribing eyeglasses, contact lenses or some other optical device. Sometimes, a vision therapy program may be recommended. Furthermore, with certain conditions, drugs may be administered by the optometrist for the treatment of eye disease.

Doctors of optometry are the only practitioners trained in all areas of optics and vision science. After completing four years of college, four years of optometry school are required for the doctor of optometry degree. In some cases, this is followed by a year of residency training in one of the optometric specialties.

The four year optometric program includes classroom education and clinical training in anatomy and physiology of the eye, ocular drugs and diseases, physiological and ophthalmic optics, visual perception and visual performance. In addition, optometrists are thoroughly trained in all areas of optics and lens design for the management of eye conditions. Other classroom training includes biochemistry, general pathology, pharmacology, endocrinology and microbiology.

Optometry schools are the only institutions where all phases of eyecare, general health sciences and optics are taught in a unified curriculum.

State optometry laws require a graduate of an optometry school to complete a three part comprehensive examination before a license is granted. In addition, optometric knowledge is assessed in a written and oral presentation as well as a practical demonstration of optometric instrumentation. Furthermore, unlike many other healthcare professionals, optometrists are required by state law to obtain a certain number of continuing education credits every year for license renewal. This is to ensure that optometric care remains at a high level and that practitioners are kept abreast of new developments in eyecare.

Optometrists, as part of the healthcare team, refer patients to other professionals, when necessary. These include medical practitioners, ophthalmologists, dermatologists, neurologists, psychologists and educators. The healthcare practitioners, ideally, work together as a team when the patient's healthcare needs are varied. Communication between professionals is necessary for the well being of the patient.

Optometry, like other areas of health care, has specializations. The basic specialties of optometry are: contact lenses, vision rehabilitation (low vision), environmental eyecare, pediatric optometry and sports vision.

The number one specialty in optometry is contact lenses. More optometrists specialize in fitting contact lenses than any of the other areas of specialization. Contact lenses can be used for cosmetic or medical reasons and very often solve vision problems which are uncorrectable by any other means. Despite their commercialization, contact lenses are a medical device and should be fitted by someone thoroughly trained in all aspects of contact lens fitting and care.

Vision rehabilitation, sometimes called low vision, is a specialty of optometry that demands a lot of interest because of the aging of the population. People with impaired vision can often be helped by sophisticated optical devices and training. Microscopic and telescopic optical systems are used to restore functional vision in patients who have some degree of usable vision. Patients who have been told that no medical solution is available are often amazed when a low vision aid improves their vision. Vision rehabilitation is the ideal specialty for optometry since it combines eye health with sophisticated optical devices.

Environmental eyecare is a relatively new specialty of optometry. Also called occupational vision, it is concerned primarily with the eyecare needs of people in their working environment. The main thrust of environmental eyecare is the avoidance of eye injuries at home and at work. The vision requirements and safety needs of the working environment are addressed by the environmental optometrist. The needs of workers range from safety eyeglasses for industrial work to prescription lenses for video display terminals.

Another specialty of optometry is pediatric eyecare. Optometrists specializing in pediatrics must be sensitive to the demands of childhood visual disorders and their treatment. Pediatric optometry is the most challenging of the optometric specialties; the diagnosis and treatment of pediatric visual disorders is complex. Care frequently involves vision therapy which can help children overcome problems with focusing, eye movement, eye coordination and perceptual skills. Vision therapy enhances the processing of visual information. Vision training exercises are also used for children with crossed-eyes and "lazy eye."

The final optometric specialty is sports vision. Sports vision includes eye safety and the improvement of athletic performance through vision training exercises. Specific sports have specific visual needs. Identifying those needs and any visual weaknesses the athlete may have is in the realm of sports vision. Many optometrists concerned with sports vision serve as consultants to sports teams and are often involved in sophisticated vision training techniques. Whether it is for the professional sports team or the weekend athlete, the goal of sports vision is to sharpen vision skills in order to enhance athletic performance.

The other two participants in eyecare are the ophthalmologist and the optician. The ophthalmologist is a medical doctor, who after four years of medical school, specializes in the diagnosis and treatment of eye diseases. The ophthalmologist receives at least three years of postgraduate training in eye surgery and medicine.

He is qualified to treat all diseases of the eye, either surgically or medically. The ophthalmologist may also diagnose refractive disorders and prescribe eyeglasses and contact lenses.

When a patient's medical condition extends beyond the scope of optometric practice, the optometrist will refer the patient to the appropriate ophthalmologist for consultation and treatment.

Similar to optometry, ophthalmology also has specializations. The majority of ophthalmologists are cataract surgeons. Other ophthalmological specialties include retinal specialists, corneal specialists, glaucoma specialists and neuro-ophthalmologists.

The optician, unlike the ophthalmologist and the optometrist, is not a doctor. An optician is a technician who grinds and dispenses eyeglasses and helps in the selection of frames. In some cases, opticians may dispense contact lenses but the contact lens fitting and eye health evaluation may only be done by an ophthalmologist or an optometrist. The optician's training is mainly concerned with making eyeglasses and frame adjustments on patients.

The Eye Examination

The Patient History

The most important part of the eye examination is the patient history. The questions that the doctor asks the patient in the beginning of the examination are more important than the diagnostic part of the exam. Very often, with proper questioning, the eye doctor will know the nature of the patient's complaint even before the testing begins.

The doctor will inquire if the patient wears glasses or contacts, how long he or she has been wearing them and for what purpose they are used. Are they worn constantly, just for reading, driving at night, computer use, etc.? The patient will be asked how long it has been since the last eye examination.

The patient will also be questioned concerning eye injuries, disease or operations. The health history of the patient must also be determined. Systemic disorders, such as hypertension and diabetes, can seriously affect the eyes. The patient's current health status and present medications are also listed on the record. Patients should always keep a handy record of their current medications and the dosage.

The health history of the patient's family is also important. The patient will be asked if there is any family history of cataracts, glaucoma, hypertension or diabetes. If there is a family history of any of these disorders, the patient is at a greater risk of developing the disorder. If there is a family history of any other ocular condition, such as retinitis pigmentosa, the patient should certainly mention it to the doctor during the history taking part of the examination.

The Chief Complaint

The eye doctor will ask the patient if they are having any difficulty or have noticed any changes in their vision. Very often, a patient will visit an eye doctor if there is a specific eye problem. This is called the chief complaint. The doctor will elaborate on the questions asked based on the chief complaint.

The following is a listing of the most common chief complaints of the eye:

- blurred distance vision
- blurred near vision
- headaches
- eyestrain
- fatigue
- eye pain
- itching

- flashes of light
- double vision
- loss of vision (few minutes)
- loss of vision (permanent)
- deviating or wandering eye
- reading difficulties
- learning problems

YOUR EYES!

- burning
- redness
- tearing
- discharge from the eye
- dry sensation
- foreign body in the eye
- spots in front of the eye
- color vision disturbances
- light sensitivity
- droopy eyelid
- protruding eye
- trauma to the eye
- halos around lights

The most common ocular complaint is blurred vision. The blurred vision may be caused by a refractive disorder such as nearsightedness (myopia), far-sightedness (hyperopia), astigmatism or presbyopia. Blurred near vision in an adult is probably presbyopia which is the inability of the lens to focus at near. Blurred near vision in a child is probably a dysfunction of the accom-modative (focusing) system of the eye.

Blurred distance vision is most likely myopia. Difficulty viewing in only dim illumination is night myopia. When the blurred vision is greater at near than at far, the condition is probably hyperopia. Astigmatism causes blur at dis-tance and at near.

Non-refractive conditions can also cause blurred vision. Transient blurred vision in a young adult may be a sign of multiple sclerosis or migraine. In an older adult, transient blurred vision may be due to carotid artery disease or other blood vessel disorders. A gradual increase in blurred vision in an adult is often a sign of a developing cataract. It may also be a sign of macular degeneration.

Headaches are another common ocular complaint. The eye doctor will question the patient concerning the description of the headache, the fre-quency, the duration, the time of onset, the location of the headache and the family history. Headaches are often caused by uncorrected refractive disor-ders. They can, at times, signal much more serious conditions such as hy-pertension, artery disease or tumors. More common causes of headaches are tension, sinus congestion or migraine.

Headaches must be investigated thoroughly. After eye conditions are ruled out, persistent headaches require an evaluation by an internist or possibly a neurologist.

Eyestrain or fatigue when reading is often a result of a dysfunction of either the accommodative or the convergence system of the eye. Difficulty with focusing or binocular vision disorders can cause vague near complaints. Generally, reading or near work will be uncomfortable and the patient will frequently avoid near tasks.

Eye pain can be either superficial or deep. Superficial eye pain is usually from a foreign object embedded in the conjuctiva or cornea. A corneal abrasion will also cause superficial, but intense, pain. Deep eye pain is caused by more serious conditions. Severe inflammations, corneal ulcers and acute glaucoma will all cause deep-seated ocular pain.

Itching and burning of the eyelids is called blepharitis and is a very common ocular complaint. An allergic conjunctivitis will also cause itching, burning eyes. Redness of the eyes is inflammation of the conjuctiva caused by either an irritation or an infection. An excessive mucous discharge is usually the sign of a bacterial infection.

Excessive tearing can be a viral conjunctivitis, a reaction to a dry eye condition or an irritation of the cornea. Excessive tearing in one eye only is usually a blocked tear duct. A dry, scratchy feeling in the eyes is another common eye problem. It is caused by either a dry eye condition where the tear production is not adequate or when there is damage to the outer layer of the cornea.

Floating strands or spots and flashes of light can range in severity from harmless vitreous floaters to a retinal detachment. The vitreous floaters or cobwebs are usually harmless debris drifting through the gel-like vitreous of the eye. A sudden onslaught of floaters may be a sign of a vitreous hemorrhage.

An occasional flashing light signals a tugging on the retina by the vitreous gel. An inordinate amount of flashing lights may indicate a detached retina. The sensation of a curtain being pulled over the eye is another sign of a detached retina.

Double vision can have numerous causes. The patient will be asked to elaborate on the double vision or diplopia. Does the double vision disappear when one eye is closed? Is the double vision horizontal or vertical; in other words is the double image side by side or one on top of the other? Is the diplopia more severe when looking in a particular direction?

Diplopia can be either monocular or binocular. Double vision in one eye (monocular) can be caused by a lens or a corneal disorder. Binocular double vision (present when both eyes are open) can be much more complicated. The misalignment of the eyes from muscle or nerve disorders will cause double vision. Binocular diplopia can be caused by eye tumors, multiple sclerosis, diabetes and strokes, to name just a few disorders. In children, the double vision is usually the result of faulty eye muscles.

Loss of vision can be transient or permanent. Transient loss of vision, such as a temporary blackout, can be a sign of an impending stroke. A sudden, permanent loss of vision in one eye may be caused by a complete blockage of the main artery to the eye.

A parent often brings a child to the eye doctor because of a deviating or wandering eye. The parent, typically, complains that the eye deviates inward. Some inward eyeturns are accompanied by farsightedness and can be helped by corrective lenses. Other eyeturns require surgery. An eyeturn, which is called strabismus, must be evaluated thoroughly to rule out a disease process and help restore binocular vision, if possible.

Reading and learning difficulties may also be the result of a visual disorder such as an uncorrected refractive condition, a disturbance in the accommodative or binocular system or a problem with information processing.

Visual information must be brought to the brain for processing and interpretation. Any breakdown from the eye to the brain to the motor system can cause a developmental or perceptual problem. The process of learning new information will be affected.

The disturbance of color vision is yet another possible complaint. Color vision problems may signal certain disease conditions but more frequently are simple genetic defects. Red-green anomalies are the most common. Genetic color vision defects almost exclusively affect males.

Increased sensitivity to light is often either an indication of a corneal disturbance such as a corneal abrasion or a viral conjunctivitis. Congenital glaucoma will also cause an increased sensitivity to light.

A droopy upper eyelid, called a ptosis, is another reason for concern. The droopy eyelid may be a sign of a muscle or nerve disorder and should be investigated. The ptosis will block vision, reduce the visual field and may present a cosmetic problem to the patient as well.

A protruding eye may be a sign of a tumor or an infection behind the eye. Both eyes protruding or bulging is often a sign of an overactive thyroid.

Trauma to the eye can cause serious damage to ocular structures and vision. Both penetrating and non-penetrating eye injuries may result in hemorrhage, swelling of ocular tissue, retinal tears, loss of intraocular pressure, fractured orbital bones, corneal damage and loss of vision.

Finally, halos around lights may result from either changes in the lens of the eye (cataract) or a rapid increase in the intraocular pressure of the eye (glaucoma attack). Rainbow halos around lights is a classic symptom of a glaucomatous attack. The condition is most prevalent at night when the pupil is largest. It is probably a result of corneal edema. Changes in the radial structure of the crystalline lens of the eye can also cause halos around lights.

The Comprehensive Examination

A comprehensive visual examination should consist of most of the following:

- patient history
- visual acuity check (reading the eye chart)
- refraction (determining the eyeglass prescription)
- testing ocular movement and binocular vision
- testing for eyeturns
- checking the accommodative and convergence systems
- checking the response of the pupils to light
- stereopsis or depth perception
- color vision
- visual field screening
- measuring the intraocular pressure
- blood pressure reading
- external evaluation of the eye
- internal evaluation of the eye, including the lens, vitreous and retina
- summary of findings and course of action

Visual Acuity

A measurement of visual acuity (reading the eye chart) is done at distance and also at near. The distance vision is first checked with no correction and then with the patient's distance correction if they are currently wearing glasses. The right eye is checked first, followed by the left eye and then both eyes together.

Eye charts with pictures or symbols are available for small children as opposed to the standard number or letter charts. Small children frequently appear to have poor visual acuity when often it is just a question of poor communication. A three year old child should have approximately 20/20 vision.

When determining visual acuity, the eye doctor will attempt to keep the testing distance and the room illumination constant. A patient's visual acuity should not change appreciably from one examiner to the next. Visual acuity findings must be accurate. They may become a legal issue such as in an insurance claim or eligibility for a driver's license.

Ocular Movement

The doctor will test for ocular movement or motility during the examination. He is assessing the integrity of the extraocular muscles and their nerves.

The most common test is the Broad H test. The patient is instructed to fixate a penlight held directly in front of his face. The doctor then moves the penlight sideways and up and down in a large H pattern instructing the patient to remain fixated on the light as it moves. The doctor is watching the patient's eyes to insure that both eyes follow the light properly in all directions of gaze.

Eyeturns

The doctor will determine if the patient has an eyeturn or eye deviation by use of the cover test. The cover test is a very simple test but gives much information. The doctor can determine if the patient has an eyeturn (in, out, up or down), which eye is deviating, if it is present at distance or at near, if it is constant and whether or not it alternates eyes.

The cover test involves an occluder which briefly covers one eye at a time and is then removed. The alternate cover test involves moving the occluder back and forth between the two eyes. The patient is fixating a target during this procedure. The doctor will be watching the eye movements during the cover test to determine if any deviation exists.

The Accommodative and Convergence Systems

In order to view an object which approaches the face, both eyes must converge inward toward the object and increase their focusing ability (accommodation). The near point of convergence is checked by slowly bringing a penlight in toward the patient's nose and asking the patient when the light goes double. The point where the penlight image splits into two is called the nearpoint of convergence. Ideally, it should be at the nose or a few inches before it.

The near point of accommodation is checked by slowly bringing a reading card in toward the patient. One eye is occluded while the other eye is being tested. The distance where the letters on the reading card blur is called the nearpoint of accommodation. As a person ages, the nearpoint of accommodation becomes further and further away until finally reading glasses are needed for near tasks.

Checking the Pupillary Response

The first pupillary check is the size of the pupil. Some people simply have pupils which are unequal in size. However, unequal pupil size may be a sign of nerve damage and should be investigated.

The doctor will then shine a bright light into each eye in order to check the pupillary response to light. Both pupils should constrict when a light is directed into one of the eyes. This so-called swinging flashlight test is a check for optic nerve disease.

Stereopsis

Stereopsis is the ability to perceive depth. In order to appreciate depth perception, both eyes must function together as a team. A common test for stereopsis is the titmus stereofly, used as a gross test on children. The child wears cross-polarized lenses while viewing a three-dimensional image of a large fly. The child is asked to reach out and touch the fly's wings, which should appear above the booklet. If the child touches the booklet, not even gross stereopsis is present.

There are more discriminating tests for stereopsis where the patient, again, wears polarized glasses to view subtle three-dimensional images. A series of targets are presented and the subject is instructed to point out which object appears to be floating above the page. A person with poor or no stereopsis will report that all of the objects appear flat. Lack of stereopsis is often from a deviated eye resulting in a loss of binocular vision.

Color Vision

Testing color vision in children, particularly males, is important for detecting congenital color defects. Congenital defects (present at birth) are usually red-green deficiencies. In adults, testing color vision is done to detect acquired color defects which may be a sign of a disease. Some retinal and optic nerve disorders can cause color vision defects later in life.

Each eye is tested separately using a plate color test held at the reading distance. Each plate has a figure consisting of dots of varying shades and brightness. The effect is to camouflage a figure from a subject having a particular defect. If the color defect is not present, the hidden figure will be visible. If the particular color defect is present, the camouflaged figure or number will not be visible. Ideally, the test should be performed in daylight illumination.

Screening the Visual Field

A comprehensive eye examination should include a screening of the patient's visual field for defects. The majority of visual field defects occur in the central visual field. Screening techniques can include automated field testers, a tangent screen or confrontations.

Confrontations consist of the doctor sitting directly across from the subject. One eye is occluded. The subject is instructed to fixate on the doctor's nose while the doctor presents fingers or other objects in different areas of the patient's visual field. The patient is asked to identify the objects or the number of fingers that are presented.

Confrontation testing is a gross assessment of the patient's central visual field. More sophisticated testing is accomplished by using a computerized (automated) visual field tester.

Measuring the Intraocular Pressure

A measurement of the intraocular pressure is one of the most important parts of the eye examination. The procedure is called tonometry. High pressure inside the eye causes damage to the optic nerve and a subsequent loss of the visual field. This condition is called glaucoma.

There are several ways to measure the intraocular pressure. A Schiotz tonometer is a small, portable instrument applied directly to an anesthetized cornea as the patient looks upward. Schiotz tonometry is called indentation tonometry since the cornea is indented during the procedure.

The other method of measuring the intraocular pressure is called applanation tonometry. Goldmann applanation tonometry involves a probe illuminated with a blue light gently touching an anesthetized cornea. It is probably the most accurate method of measuring the intraocular pressure. Other applanation methods include Mackay Marg tonometry where a probe is tapped several times against the cornea and the non-contact tonometer where a puff of air is directed at the cornea.

All of the methods measure the eye pressure in millimeters of mercury (mm Hg). Normal pressure readings range from 10 mm Hg to 20 mm Hg Readings of 21 mm Hg or higher are suspicious and should be repeated on a different day or investigated further.

Blood Pressure

Most comprehensive eye exams today also include a check of the patient's blood pressure. High blood pressure and its complications is the leading cause of death in the United States today. Along with heart, artery and kidney problems, high blood pressure (hypertension) can also affect the eyes. Severe or prolonged hypertension can cause damage to retinal blood vessels and threaten vision.

When blood pressure readings are elevated, the optometrist will refer the patient to his internist for appropriate treatment.

External Evaluation of the Eye

The doctor will use a biomicroscope or slit lamp for evaluation of the external parts of the eye. The biomicroscope magnifies and illuminates the viewed object.

The doctor will first check the quality and quantity of the tears. The lids and lid margins will then be checked for infections or growths. The cornea and conjuctiva will then be evaluated. The iris, sclera, lens and anterior chamber of the eye can also be checked with a biomicroscope without the use of special lenses.

Internal Evaluation of the Eye

A comprehensive eye examination must include a total assessment of the internal health of the eye. A dilated evaluation is more complete since it allows the peripheral retina to be viewed. An ophthalmoscope, either a hand held ophthalmoscope or a binocular indirect ophthalmoscope, is used for examining the internal structures of the eye. The internal evaluation will

YOUR EYES!

include an examination of the lens of the eye, the vitreous gel, the optic nerve, the macula and the peripheral retina.

Special lenses are required for examining the internal eye, either with or without a biomicroscope. The evaluation of the internal structures of the eye is usually performed at the end of the eye examination.

2

Anatomy of the Eye

The Eyelids

The major function of the eyelids is to protect the eye. This is accomplished in three ways: the eyelashes help keep particles out of the eye, glands under the eyelid secrete substances which lubricate the eye and movement of the lids help to protect the eye from injury.

The eyelashes act as a screen to filter particles and help keep the eye free of debris. The eyelashes (cilia) are located on the lid margins. There are about 150 lashes on the upper lid and about 70 on the lower lid. The upper lid lashes are curved up and outward and the lower lid lashes are curved down and outward. Just a very gentle touch of a lash will trigger the blink reflex and the eye will protectively close.

The base of each lash is surrounded by an oil secreting gland called a Zeis gland. Infection of this gland results in a stye. If a lash is pulled out, a new one will replace it in about 8 weeks.

Secretions of eyelid glands form the next system of protection. Meibomian glands, which are large oil secreting glands in the lid, help produce the oily

YOUR EYES!

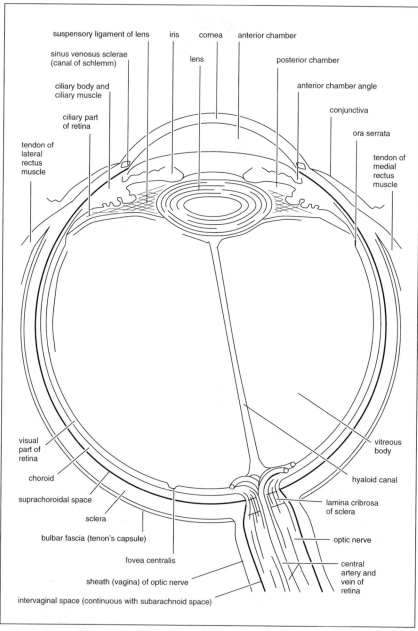

The human eye.

layer of the tears. The oily layer of the tears is the outer layer and this prevents the evaporation of the tears. There are about 30 of these glands in each lid. They are oriented perpendicular to the lid margin forming a single row at the margin. Squeezing the lid margin will produce sebum oozing out of the glands.

Aqueous and mucous producing glands are also located in the eyelids. These glands also contribute to the tear film.

The major protective mechanism of the lids is their ability for quick movement. The elevation of the upper eyelid is due to stimulation by the third cranial nerve to the levator palpebral muscle located in the upper eyelid. When the levator is stimulated, the upper lid can be raised about 10 mm.

The orbicularis oculi muscle (innervated by cranial nerve VII) closes the eye. Closing the eye (blinking) can be either spontaneous or forceful. Spontaneous blinking occurs at frequent intervals during waking hours and its purpose is to help keep the cornea lubricated with tears.

The blink rate varies depending on the mental state of the individual; excitement increases the blink rate and intense concentration lowers it. The average person blinks about 15 times a minute. Despite the fact that vision is briefly interrupted when blinking, the sensation of vision remains continuous.

Forceful blinking (reflex blinking) is a reaction to a particular stimuli. A bright light, a quick movement of an object toward the eye or loud noises will all cause a quick forceful closing of the eyes as a protective mechanism.

Any object touching the cornea will produce a blink reflex. First time contact lens wearers can attest to this.

The dazzle reflex can be produced by shining a very bright light into the eye, causing a forceful blink. Sometimes, a bright light shining in the eye can produce a sneeze reflex. Strange as it may seem, some people actually sneeze when first going outdoors in bright sunlight.

The Cornea

The cornea is a transparent living tissue, lacking blood vessels, which covers the outer part of the eye. It approximately covers the iris, about 12 millimeters in diameter. The cornea is about 1 mm thick in the periphery and about 0.5 mm thick in the center.

YOUR EYES!

The cornea is a powerful refractive surface allowing light rays to pass unimpeded to the retina. It bends the light sufficiently to allow proper focusing.

The cornea also acts as a protective membrane; it is a barrier to microorganisms as long as the membrane remains intact. If the barrier is broken, serious infections can then result.

The cornea becomes swollen after the eyes have been closed for a period of time, such as during sleep. Fluid retention (edema) causes the increased thickness. After the eyes are opened, the air dehydrates the cornea reducing its thickness.

The cornea is composed of 5 layers: the epithelium, Bowman's membrane, the stroma, Descemet's membrane and the endothelium.

The epithelium is the outermost layer forming a uniform thickness and regularity. The epithelial cells form a smooth surface which is compatible with the tear layer.

Bowman's membrane is a sheet of tough, transparent tissue consisting mostly of collagen material, running parallel to the surface. It does not contain any cells.

The corneal stroma is composed of layers of tissue called lamellae which extend the entire length of the cornea. The lamellae are attached loosely to each other. About 90% of the cornea is composed of stromal tissue. The stroma has cell bodies called keratocytes which are interlaced with one another.

The fourth layer is called Descemet's membrane. It is secretory products from the innermost layer, the endothelium.

The endothelium is a single layer of cells pressed up against Descemet's membrane. Endothelial cells cannot reproduce and their quantity and quality decrease over time. As endothelial cells die, the remaining cells enlarge and spread over Descemet's membrane to keep it completely covered.

When either the epithelium or endothelium is damaged, swelling of stromal tissue develops. Indeed, any damage to the integrity of the cornea can lead to localized swelling.

The corneal epithelium regenerates quickly and the healing process is rapid. Since endothelial cells do not regenerate, endothelial damage is much more serious. Permanent swelling and loss of transparency may result.

The epithelium and endothelium act as fluid barriers and their integrity is essential in order to maintain the proper dehydrated state. When the barrier is broken, fluid builds up in the stroma and the cornea loses its transparency.

The endothelium acts as a chemical pump; removing water and sodium from the stroma. As long as the pump is maintained, fluid will not build up and the cornea will remain clear.

The corneal epithelium has a rich supply of nerve fibers, supplied by the fifth cranial nerve called the trigeminal nerve. Whenever the nerve fibers are exposed, severe pain results. The large amount of nerves and their proximity to the surface make even minor corneal injuries quite painful.

The sources of the cornea's nutrition are the limbal blood vessels surrounding the cornea and the atmosphere, which supplies some oxygen to the superficial cornea. Since the cornea has no blood vessels, nutritional elements pass to the cornea through the limbus. The limbus is the junction between the cornea and the sclera.

The Conjuctiva

The conjuctiva is a thin, transparent mucous membrane that covers the underside of the lids (palpebral conjuctiva) and the front surface of the sclera (bulbar conjuctiva).

The palpebral conjuctiva is firmly attached to the underside of the lid. The bulbar conjuctiva is attached to the sclera which is seen as the white of the eye through the transparent conjuctiva.

The bulbar conjuctiva is loosely attached to the orbital wall and this permits the eye to move freely.

The blood supply to the palpebral conjuctiva comes from the arterial arcades of the eyelid. The bulbar conjuctiva receives its blood supply from peripheral branches which are superficial and nearly invisible. When an inflammation affects the conjunctiva (conjunctivitis), it is the bulbar conjunctival blood vessels that appear bright red.

The conjunctival epithelium contains many mucous producing glands. The mucous is the wetting agent of the tear film; it allows proper wetting of the corneal epithelium by the tears.

Because it is the outermost tissue of the eye, the conjunctiva is exposed to many microorganisms and irritating substances. The tears help fight off microorganisms by diluting them and also by producing chemicals which help reduce bacterial growth.

A conjunctivitis is marked by red, swollen conjunctiva with excess tearing, gummy lids in the morning and possibly increased light sensitivity. Besides microorganisms, irritating substances can also cause a conjunctivitis. Smoke, wind and pollution can all cause the classic red eye appearance.

The Lacrimal System

The lacrimal system consists of the lacrimal gland, puncta, canaliculi, tear sac and the nasolacrimal duct. The lacrimal system produces and eliminates the tears.

The lacrimal gland, which produces the tears, is located in the upper, temple side of the orbit. The tears flow through ducts down to the cornea and bulbar and palpebral conjunctiva. These structures are moistened by the tears.

The tears then drain through the puncta into the canaliculi which are little channels about 8 mm long. The puncta are tiny holes located on the medial part of both upper and lower lids. A punctum can be observed by pulling the lower lid slightly and noting the tiny hole on the margin of the lid towards the nose.

The lacrimal canaliculi join to form a common canaliculus before opening into the lacrimal sac. The lacrimal sac drains down into the bony nasolacrimal duct. The duct empties behind the nose and nasopharynx and down into the throat. This is why after inserting some types of eye drops, the patient can taste the medication. The drops flow with the tears down into the throat.

The Orbit

The orbit is a bony cavity of four walls which holds the eyeball and adjacent structures. The four walls converge posteriorly. The inside walls of the right and left orbit are parallel and are separated by the nose.

The orbit is surrounded by the sinuses; the frontal sinus above, the maxillary sinus below and the ethmoid and sphenoid sinuses on the inside.

The orbital wall is very thin and is easily damaged by trauma to the eye. A "blowout" fracture results when the orbital floor is cracked and the orbital contents may protrude downward.

The eyeball occupies only about 20% of the orbital space. The remaining orbital space is filled with fat and muscle.

The main artery supplying the orbit and its contents is the ophthalmic artery which is the first major branch of the internal carotid artery. Superior and inferior veins drain the blood from the orbit. All the nerves and blood vessels supplying the eye enter at the apex of the orbit. The apex is also the origin of all of the extraocular muscles except the inferior oblique.

The anterior part of the orbit is the only open area. Any increase in orbital contents will, therefore, push the eyeball forward since this is the only direction that it can expand. A protruding eyeball is called proptosis and it can result from any space occupying lesion or swelling inside the orbit.

Sphenoid and ethmoid sinus infections can erode the inner wall of the orbit leading to involvement of the orbital contents.

Orbital cellulitis is a serious infection of the orbital contents. The eyelids swell and become red and pain will be present with eye movement. There may be fever and the infection can spread beyond the orbit causing a life-threatening situation. It is treated aggressively with antibiotics.

The Lens

The lens of the eye is a biconvex, almost transparent structure about 4mm thick and about 9 mm long. It is suspended behind the iris. In front of the lens is the aqueous, behind it is the vitreous.

The lens contains a nucleus, cortex and a capsule. The lens capsule is a semi-permeable membrane encasing the lens which allows water and minerals to pass through.

The nucleus and cortex are made of long, concentric lamellar fibers. The nucleus is harder than the cortex. The fibers are continuously being produced and directed inward as a person ages. This is why the lens loses its elasticity in later life reducing its ability to change shape easily (accommodation). This makes focusing on near objects difficult and necessitates the need for reading glasses or bifocals.

The lens is composed of 35% protein and 65% water with a trace of body minerals. There are no nerves or blood vessels in the lens. Nutrition is obtained from the surrounding fluids: the vitreous and the aqueous. Chemical energy from glucose allows the lens to maintain its transparency and continue to grow throughout life.

The lens refracts light entering the eye through the pupil and allows it to properly focus on the retina. If the lens is removed because of a cataract, the refractive power must be replaced. Either an intraocular implant, a contact lens or thick eyeglasses must be substituted to restore the lost refractive power.

Besides contributing to part of the refractive power of the eye and providing accommodation when needed, another important feature of the lens is its ability to absorb ultraviolet radiation. Ultraviolet radiation from the environment is prevented from reaching the retina by the lens proteins.

Absorption of ultraviolet radiation by the lens leads to discoloration of lens tissue. Any breakdown of the transparency of the lens, either an opacity or discoloration, is a cataract. Studies have shown that people who work outdoors or who are exposed to long periods of bright sunlight have a higher incidence of cataracts compared to the general population. This applies to patients over the age of 65, but everyone would do well by guarding against too much ultraviolet exposure.

The Pupil

The pupil is the center opening of the iris. The amount of light entering the eye is regulated by constriction of the pupil in bright light and dilation of the pupil in dim light. The iris muscles control the pupil size.

Pupils are normally round with a regular shape and are very similar in size. The pupil is actually located just slightly below center and slightly towards the nose. When the left and right pupils are different sizes, the condition is called anisocoria.

Pupil size varies throughout life. It is smallest in infancy and old age and is largest during adolescence.

When a person becomes excited, the pupils will dilate. Certain drugs, such as amphetamines, also cause dilation of the pupils. The pupils will also enlarge in darkness or dim illumination.

The pupils constrict when exposed to bright illumination and also during sleep and when looking at near objects. Some drugs, the opiates for example, will also cause the pupils to constrict.

When a penlight is directed into one eye, both pupils will constrict. This is called the light reflex. This occurs because the optic nerve fibers from both eyes cross each other and have a common nucleus. When optic nerve damage is present, a bright light directed into the affected eye will not cause the pupils to constrict. When an eye doctor shines his penlight into your eyes, he is checking the pupillary response to rule out optic nerve disease.

A somewhat uncommon pupillary condition is called Adie's Syndrome. One pupil reacts poorly to light and stays relatively dilated when a bright light is directed into the affected eye. It also constricts poorly when viewing near objects. There is no apparent nerve damage present to explain the condition.

It typically occurs in females, age 20 to 40, and almost always occurs in only one eye. The condition is sometimes referred to as Adie's tonic pupil. The onset is abrupt and the main symptom is blurred near vision since a normal eye will constrict when viewing near objects to allow focusing. Reading glasses are sometimes prescribed.

For some unexplained reason, 90% of patients with Adie's tonic pupil will have a diminished knee jerk reflex. When the doctor taps the knee during a physical examination, the knee jerk will be reduced.

The cause of Adie's tonic pupil appears to be a slow-acting, benign virus which affects the nerve bundle. There is no explanation, however, for the loss of the knee jerk reflex.

The Extraocular Muscles

Eye movements are controlled by the extraocular muscles. Each eye has six muscles attached to it: the lateral rectus, the medial rectus, the inferior rectus, the superior rectus, the superior oblique and the inferior oblique. These muscles, either alone or working together, are responsible for every possible eye movement.

The lateral rectus muscle arises from the posterior apex of the orbit and runs forward along the outside of the globe and attaches to the sclera about 7 mm from the border of the cornea. It is supplied by the sixth cranial nerve. The sole function of the lateral rectus muscle is to turn the eye outward.

The medial rectus also starts at the posterior apex of the orbit and runs forward along the inside of the globe and attaches to the sclera about 6 mm from the border of the cornea. It is the thickest and most powerful of the extraocular muscles and has a very short tendon. The medial rectus is supplied by a branch of the third cranial nerve. The sole function of the medial rectus is to turn the eye inward.

The inferior rectus muscle arises from the posterior apex of the orbit and runs forward beneath the globe and attaches to the sclera about 6 mm from the border of the cornea. It is also supplied by the third cranial nerve.

The inferior rectus muscle has several functions. Its main function is depressing the globe allowing the eye to look downward. Its secondary actions help the eye turn inward and also help to rotate it.

The superior rectus muscle also arises from the posterior apex of the orbit and runs forward above the globe and attaches to the sclera about 8 mm from the border of the cornea. It is supplied by a branch of the third cranial nerve. The superior rectus muscle travels with the levator palpebral muscle which is responsible for elevating the eyelid.

The superior rectus also has several functions. Its primary function is to elevate the globe allowing the eye to look upward. Its secondary actions help the eye turn inward and also help to rotate it.

The superior oblique muscle begins just above the posterior apex of the orbit and runs forward above and towards the inner side of the eyeball. It then reaches a U-shaped pulley called the trochlea which is attached to the bony orbit. The muscle goes through the U-shaped pulley and turns sharply backward over the globe to insert into the sclera at the globe's equator. The superior oblique muscle is supplied by the fourth cranial nerve. The primary function of the superior oblique muscle is to rotate the eyeball inward.

The remaining extraocular muscle is the inferior oblique. Unlike the other extraocular muscles, the inferior oblique arises from the floor of the orbit and not the posterior apex of the orbit. It passes backward, not forward, and inserts on the globe on the outer side just below the lateral rectus muscle. It is supplied by a branch of the third cranial nerve. The primary function of the inferior oblique muscle is to rotate the eyeball outward.

Hering's Law

When the eyes are directed into a field of gaze (both eyes looking to the right, for example), they must turn an equal amount in order to maintain binocular vision. Non-corresponding muscles of each eye must be activated. Hering's Law states that, with all voluntary eye movements, both eyes will receive equal, simultaneous nerve stimulation. Equal nerve stimulation results in both eyes moving equal amounts.

As an example, when looking to the right, the right lateral rectus muscle is stimulated which turns the right eye outward. At the same time, the left medial rectus muscle is also equally stimulated. This turns the left eye inward. The end result (because of equal stimulation) is both eyes looking to the right and maintaining a single image.

Neuroanatomy

The Visual Pathway

The optic nerve is a trunk containing about one million nerve axons arising from the ganglion cells of the retina. The nerve emerges through the back of the globe through a circular opening in the sclera. The nerve travels through the orbit, about 25 mm, then passes through the bony optic canal into the cranial cavity. After another 10 mm, the nerve joins the opposite optic nerve to form the optic chiasm. *(Figure 2-1)*

At the optic chiasm, axons from the nasal retina of the opposite side and axons from the temporal retina of the same side form the optic tracts. The optic tracts lead to the lateral geniculate body where the retinal axons carrying visual impulses synapse. The lateral geniculate body modifies the strength of the retinal signal. It has been suggested that the lateral geniculate body also plays a role in color vision and depth perception.

The axons continue from the lateral geniculate body to form the optic radiations. The optic radiations terminate in the visual cortex which is located in the posterior part of the brain called the occipital lobe. Here the visual information is processed and integrated with visual information from the other side of the brain.

The Visual Field

The normal visual field is as follows: laterally 85 degrees, nasally 60 degrees, up 45 degrees and down 65 degrees. This is the visual field for each eye. *(Figure 2-2)* The nasal retina (the inner part of the retina towards the nose) projects the visual field temporally (outside). The temporal retina (the outer part of the retina towards the temple) projects the visual field nasally (inside). *(Figure 2-3)*

Damage to the nasal retina results in a temporal visual field loss and damage to the temporal retina results in a nasal visual field loss. If the optic nerve is severed, the eye will be totally blind.

If damage is done to one of the optic tracts or optic radiations, a visual field defect called an homonymous hemianopia develops. If the right optic tract

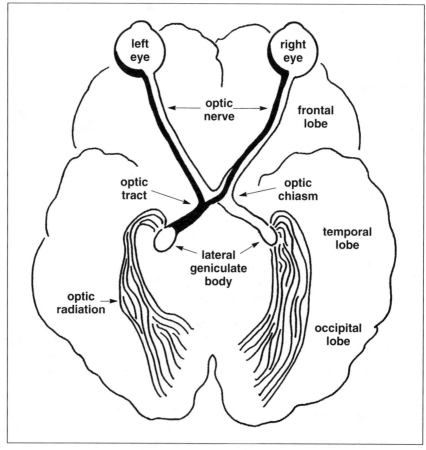

Figure 2-1 The visual pathway.

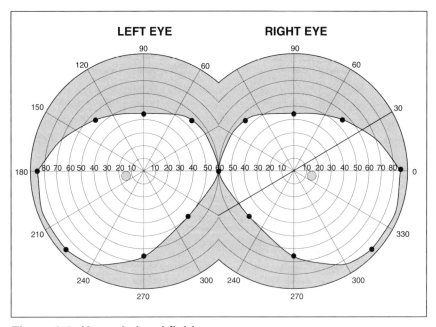

Figure 2-2   Normal visual field.

or radiation is destroyed, a left homonymous hemianopia develops; the left visual field of each eye is lost. If the left optic tract or radiation is destroyed a right homonymous hemianopia develops; the right visual field of each eye is lost. *(Figure 2-4)*

Very often, field defects of this nature can result from a stroke. A stroke on the left side of the brain will cause problems on the right side of the body. A stroke on the left side of the brain will, therefore, cause a right-side visual field defect.

The Blind Spot

The blind spot is the point where the optic nerve leaves the back of the eye. At this location of the retina, there are no photoreceptors and hence no vision. With normal vision, the blind spot is not noticed because the brain tunes it out. *(See the demonstration of the blind spot in Figure 2-5)*

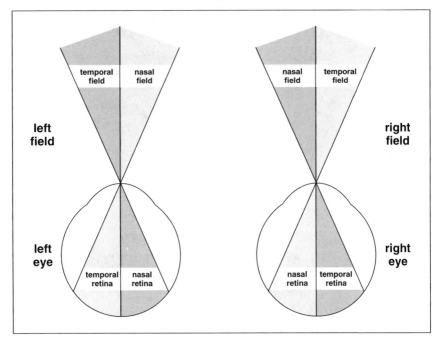

Figure 2-3 Temporal retina sees nasal field and nasal retina sees temporal field.

The Cranial Nerves

The cranial nerves involved with vision and the eye are cranial nerves: II, III, IV, V, VI and VII.

The Optic Nerve is cranial nerve II and it brings the visual image from the retinal ganglion cells eventually to the brain for processing.

The Oculomotor Nerve is cranial nerve III. The Oculomotor Nerve supplies the inferior oblique muscle, the inferior, superior and medial recti muscles and the levator palpebral muscle. It is also responsible for constricting the pupil, allowing the eye to focus on near objects. Damage to cranial nerve III causes a fixed, dilated pupil that cannot respond to light. The upper lid will droop (ptosis) and the eye will turn down and outward.

A sudden onset of a third nerve palsy is a medical emergency since an aneurysm of the carotid artery is a possible cause. Other causes include trauma and diabetes.

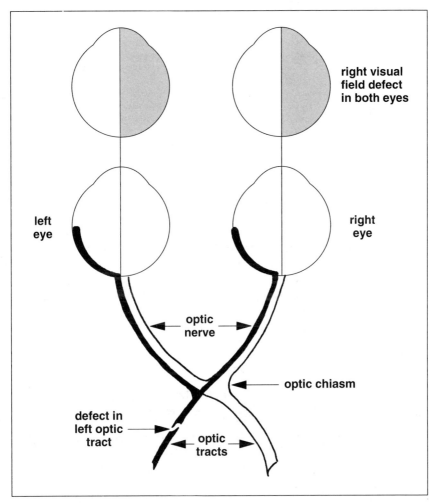

right visual
field defect
in both eyes

left
eye

right
eye

optic
nerve

optic chiasm

defect in
left optic
tract

optic
tracts

Figure 2-4 Defect in left optic tract causes right visual field defect in both eyes.

The Trochlear Nerve is cranial nerve IV. The Trochlear Nerve supplies the superior oblique muscle which rotates the eye inward.

The Trigeminal Nerve is cranial nerve V. The Trigeminal Nerve is the sensory nerve for the face and head. Sensory nerves go to the brain to supply information. Motor nerves go from the brain to respond to that information. The ophthalmic branch of the Trigeminal Nerve supplies the eye and the

Figure 2-5 **The blind spot: Close your left eye and stare, with your right eye, at the cross on this page. Hold the book at normal reading distance. While staring at the cross, the dark spot on the right side should not be visible (you may have to move the page slightly to make it disappear). This is the blind spot for the right eye and it is located about 15 degrees to the right of center.**

surrounding area. A sensation of pain in the eye, for example, is relayed to the brain via the Trigeminal Nerve.

The Abducens Nerve is cranial nerve VI. The Abducens Nerve supplies the lateral rectus muscle which turns the eye outward.

The Facial Nerve is cranial nerve VII. The Facial Nerve is the motor nerve for the eye and face. It supplies the facial muscles responsible for movement. Any action of the facial muscles, including closing the eye, is from a response of the Facial Nerve.

The Sclera

The sclera is the white, outer protective coating of the eye. It is continuous with the cornea anteriorly and with the sheath of the optic nerve posteriorly. It is about 1 mm thick and is composed of dense, fibrous material. The sclera is penetrated by arteries, veins and nerves supplying the internal eye.

The outer surface of the sclera is covered by the episclera which is a thin layer of elastic tissue. The episclera contains blood vessels that nourish the sclera.

Underneath the sclera is the pigmented uveal tract. Certain connective tissue disorders can thin the normally white sclera and the sclera then develops a bluish discoloration as the underlying pigment is exposed. Prolonged use of steroids can also cause a blue sclera. Normal, healthy newborns may also have a bluish appearance to their sclera.

Inflammation of the sclera is called scleritis and inflammation of the episclera is called episcleritis. The symptoms of both include: pain, redness, light sensitivity and excessive tearing. There are many possible causes of a scleritis or an episcleritis. Some of the more common are rheumatoid arthritis, herpes and gout. Radiation and chemical burns can also cause inflammed scleral tissue.

The most common injury to the sclera is from trauma, either from a blunt trauma or a penetrating injury. Flying objects can penetrate the dense, fibrous tissue of the sclera resulting in an intraocular hemorrhage and damage to internal structures.

The Uveal Tract

The uveal tract is composed of three pigmented parts: the iris, the ciliary body and the choroid.

The iris is the anterior extension of the ciliary body and the ciliary body is the anterior extension of the choroid. The three structures together are called the uveal tract and it is considered the middle layer of the eye. The uveal tract is covered by the cornea and the sclera.

The most anterior section of the uveal tract is the iris. The iris is a flat, muscular surface with a round opening in the center called the pupil. The iris contacts the lens posteriorly and the aqueous anteriorly. The aqueous is the fluid in the anterior chamber of the eye.

The muscles of the iris are called the sphincter and dilator muscles. The sphincter muscle constricts the pupil and the dilator muscle dilates or opens the pupil.

The iris is attached to the ciliary body which is the middle portion of the uveal tract. The ciliary body contains muscles which are attached to zonular fibers which are, in turn, attached to the lens. The function of the ciliary muscle is to contract or relax the zonular fibers. This alters the tension on the lens and allows the lens to change focus.

Another part of the ciliary body, called ciliary processes, produce the aqueous fluid.

The most posterior part of the uveal tract is the choroid. The choroid is the middle layer of the eye and lies between the retina and the sclera. It has a very large supply of blood vessels, and its main function is to nourish the retina.

Inflammation of the uveal tract is called uveitis. It is characterized by pain, light sensitivity and blurred vision. The eye may become red and the pupil usually becomes small. In most cases, a cause cannot be found. Steroids are given to reduce the inflammation and help alleviate the symptoms.

The Vitreous

The vitreous is a clear, gel-like substance that fills the posterior cavity of the eye. It forms a support framework for the retina. Light penetrates the vitreous quite easily and nutrients diffuse through the vitreous to the retina.

The vitreous fills a volume of about 4 milliliters and its water content is about 99%. The framework of the vitreous is composed of collagen fibers. The vitreous is firmly attached to the optic nerve, part of the ciliary body and the peripheral retina.

When the vitreous shrinks and pulls away from the retina, this is called a posterior vitreous detachment. Posterior vitreous detachments are quite common, in fact, several studies suggest that they occur in about 70% of patients over the age of 65.

Usually, the vitreous pulls away cleanly. However, in some cases, a retinal tear can develop from a posterior vitreous detachment and can lead to a retinal detachment. A retinal detachment is an ocular emergency.

The symptoms of a posterior vitreous detachment and a retinal detachment are the same: flashing lights and/or suddenly appearing floaters which may resemble flys or spiders. When these symptoms are present, a complete ocular examination including dilation, is warranted.

The Retina

The retina is the innermost coat of the eye containing light sensitive nerve tissue. If the eye is a camera, the retina is the film.

The anatomy of the retina is quite complex. The retina consists of ten layers: from the most posterior layer, Bruch's membrane, to the most anterior internal limiting membrane adjacent to the vitreous.

The retina covers the inner part of the back two-thirds wall of the globe. It is a multi-layered sheet of nerve tissue attached to a pigmented epithelium. The pigmented layer is attached to Bruch's membrane.

The retina is about 0.20 mm thick and is thinnest at the center of the macula (fovea centralis). The retinal tissue is transparent, except for the retinal blood vessels. When viewing the posterior pole of the eye, it is the pigmented layer that is visible, attached to the transparent retina in front of it.

The rods and cones are the photoreceptors of the eye; in the fovea all of the photoreceptors are cones. As the peripheral retina is approached, more of the photoreceptors are rods and less are cones. There are about 6 million cones and 100 million rods in the retina. The optic nervehead has no photoreceptors. The area responsible for color vision covers about 9 mm and is centered at the fovea.

The cones are responsible for color vision and fine visual discrimination. The rods are responsible for motion detection and night vision.

The retina has no pain nerve fibers, therefore, retinal diseases are painless.

The retina receives its blood supply from two separate sources. The outer third of the retina receives its blood supply from capillaries attached to the outer part of Brach's membrane. The inner two-thirds of the retina receives its blood supply from branches of the central retinal artery.

The axons of the photoreceptor cells pass directly to the outer plexiform layer where they eventually connect to the inner nuclear layer and then on to the ganglion cell layer. The long axons of the ganglion cells become the optic nerve where the nerve impulse is transmitted, via the visual pathway, to the brain for processing.

YOUR EYES!

3

How the Eye Functions In Vision

I. Optics

Through the ages, there have been many distorted theories attempting to explain how we see the world around us. One very early theory suggested that the eyes send out rays of light illuminating what we see. Another erroneous concept of vision suggested that objects gave off color.

What actually happens is that light comes into the eye from surrounding objects. Light is energy emitted in waves or rays. The light travels 186,000 miles a second, when measured in a vacuum. Generally, light travels in a straight line.

In order to provide a sharp image on the retina, these light rays entering the eye must be bent. The cornea and the lens of the eye help bend the light rays permitting proper focus on the retina. The rays entering the eye from an angle are said to be refracted.

Light rays can either be divergent, convergent or parallel. A light source always emits diverging rays. A convergent or parallel wave results when diverging rays reach a limiting aperture or opening, such as the pupil. The light rays entering the center part of the pupil go straight back to the retina. The light rays entering the peripheral part of the pupil are bent to allow focusing on the retina. *(Figure 3-1)*

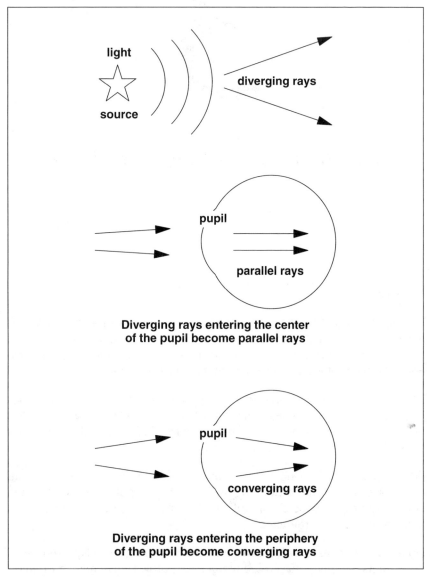

Figure 3-1 Diverging light rays.

The eye behaves somewhat like a pinhole camera. Rays of light pass through the pupil (aperture) in a straight line striking the retina (film). Each ray of light passes through the pupil independently and forms a tiny patch of light on the retina. If the retinal image could be caught on a screen, it would be inverted (upside down) and proportional to the object being viewed. *(Figure 3-2)*

Light travels in waves with specific distances between the waves called wavelengths. The wavelengths are measured in nanometers (0.0000001 meter). The waves contain energy; the shorter the wavelength, the higher the energy.

The limits of visible light are between 390 nm and 760 nm Below 390 nm and above 760 nm, energy waves are not visible to the human eye. An example of an energy wave below 390 nm is ultraviolet light and an example of an energy wave above 760 nm is a radio wave. All of the colors of the spectrum fall between 390 nm and 760 nm.

When white light strikes a prism, the colors of the visible spectrum are produced. A prism is a transparent structure that deviates light. *(Figures 3-3 and 3-4)*

The colors have specific wavelengths and energy levels. As the colors strike the retina, the visual effects vary from a sensation of red (longest wavelength) to a sensation of violet (shortest wavelength). The color red has the least amount of energy and the color violet has the highest energy level.

Like prisms, lenses also bend light. A convex lens will converge light and a concave lens will diverge light. A convex lens (a plus lens) is used to correct

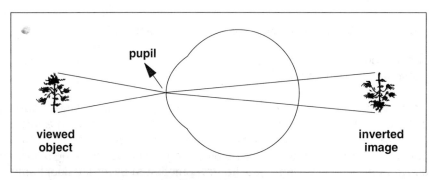

Figure 3-2 The eye as a pinhole camera.

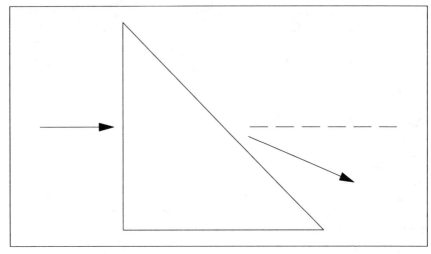

Figure 3-3 Prism deviating light ray.

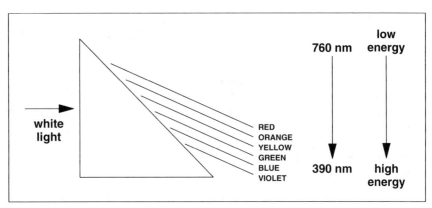

Figure 3-4 Prism dispersing colors of the spectrum.

farsightedness. A concave lens (a minus lens) is used to correct near-sightedness. *(Figures 3-5 and 3-6)*

Convex and concave lenses, worn as eyeglasses, can sometimes cause distortion, particularly with high prescriptions. A person wearing a thick, concave lens, when viewing a door frame, sometimes notices the frame bends outward like a barrel. On the other hand, a person wearing a thick, convex lens, when viewing a door frame, sometimes notices the door frame bends inward like a pincushion. Both effects usually diminish with time.

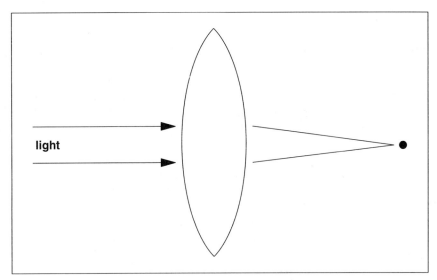

Figure 3-5 Convex lens converges light rays to a point.

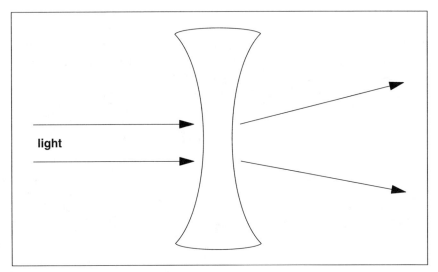

Figure 3-6 Concave lens diverges light rays.

Another effect of lenses is the alteration of the retinal image size. Convex lenses magnify images and concave lenses minify or shrink images. A high prescription (either convex or concave) for a first-time wearer requires a period of adjustment. To the convex lens wearer, objects may appear noticeably larger and the concave lens wearer may notice objects appearing smaller. The magnification and minification effects are not as dramatic with contact lenses and the visual adjustment is usually minimal.

The refractive power of a lens, the ability to deviate light, is measured in diopters (D). One diopter is the strength of a lens needed to focus parallel light rays at a distance of one meter. A one diopter lens has a focal length of one meter. *(Figure 3-7)*

The dioptric power can also be expressed as the inverse of the focal length. The higher the dioptric power, the greater the convergence of the rays and the shorter the focal length. A 5D lens, for example, has a focal length of only 20 centimeters (1/5 = 0.2 meter = 20 centimeters).

The amount of deviation through a prism is also expressed in diopters, called prism diopters. A prism with one prism diopter will deviate light one centimeter at a distance of one meter. *(Figure 3-8)*

The human eye has the total refractive power of about 60 diopters. This is the total amount of deviation as a light ray entering the eye passes through the cornea, aqueous, lens and vitreous before focusing on the retina. When the retina is 22.22 millimeters (0.022 meter) behind the refractive surface of a 60D eye and the image is focused directly on the retina, the eye is emmetropic (having no refractive error). The focal point falls on the retina.

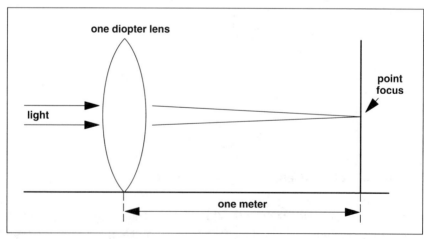

Figure 3-7 The diopter.

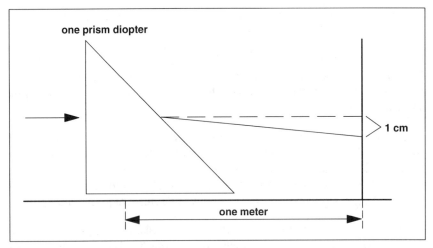

one prism diopter

1 cm

one meter

Figure 3-8 The prism diopter.

If the focal point falls in front of the retina, the eye is myopic or nearsighted. If the focal point falls behind the retina, the eye is hyperopic or farsighted.

Similarly, an eye that is unusually long (greater than 22 millimeters in length) will be nearsighted because the focal point will fall in front of the retina. An eye that is unusually short (less than 22 millimeters in length) will be farsighted because the focal point will fall behind the retina.

II. Physiology of Vision

The Photochemistry of the Retina

The retina's unique function is visual excitation. The retina absorbs light energy and, through a series of chemical reactions, converts the light into electrical nerve impulses. The process is complex and not completely understood.

The retina is a living tissue, and like all living things, requires nutrients for energy production. The main fuel for the retina, as well as the rest of the body, is glucose (blood sugar). The glucose and tremendous amounts of oxygen help fuel the high metabolic rate of the retina.

Retinal tissue dies very quickly when the oxygen supply is blocked. A central retinal artery occlusion is a blockage of the main artery of the retina and is, obviously, a medical emergency. As the oxygen supply is choked off, the retinal tissue withers and dies and the vision is destroyed.

The photoreceptors of the retina are the rods and cones. These light sensitive cells trap the light energy entering the eye. The energy is then converted into electrical energy which is rapidly transmitted to the brain via the visual pathway.

This conversion of energy is accomplished by a series of photo-chemical reactions. Vitamin A (also called retinol) triggers the photochemical reaction in the rods. The rods are the receptors responsible for night vision. The retina requires a continuous supply of Vitamin A and a person who is deprived of Vitamin A for a significant period of time will develop night blindness.

The photoreceptors contain light sensitive cells called visual pigments. The rod visual pigment is called rhodopsin and recently the three cone visual pigments were discovered. The cone visual pigments are responsible for color vision.

The three types of cone visual pigments are: blue sensitive cones, green sensitive cones, and red sensitive cones. The blue sensitive cones respond to the color blue which has a wavelength of about 450 nm. The green sensitive cones respond to the color green which has a wavelength of about 525 nm. And the red sensitive cones respond to the color red which has a wavelength of about 555 nm.

Light in dim illumination stimulates the rods and light in bright illumination stimulates the cones. The visual pigment in the photoreceptors then converts the light energy into elctrochemical energy which triggers a nerve impulse. The nerve impulse travels from the ganglion cells in the retina to the optic nerve and, through the visual pathway, to the brain for processing.

The transformation of energy is from light energy to chemical energy to electrical nerve impulses.

The Electroretinogram (ERG)

The light stimulated retinal response can be measured by taking an electroretinogram. The electroretinogram measures the electrical impulses in the retina. The principle is the same as an EKG which measures the electrical impulses in the heart and an EEG which measures the electrical impulses in the brain.

In dim illumination, a response of the rods is elicited called a scotopic response and in bright illumination, a response of the cones is elicited called a photopic response. *(Figure 3-9)*

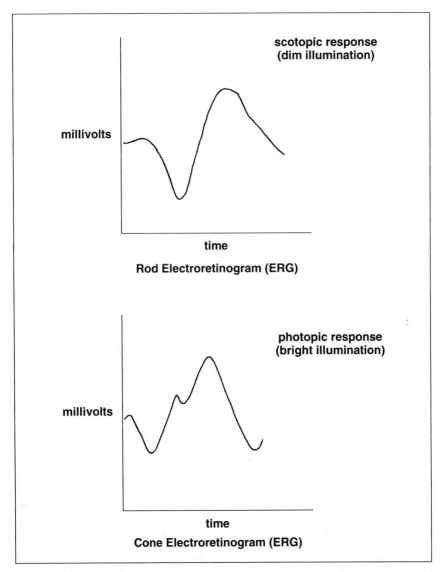

Figure 3-9 The electroretinogram

Electrodes are attached to the patient; a contact lens electrode is placed over the cornea and a reference electrode is placed on the skin over the cheekbone. Flashes of light are presented to the patient for brief intervals and a recording device measures the electrical response of the retina.

The electroretinogram is an important diagnostic tool. Certain retinal disorders give characteristic electroretinograms. Retinitis Pigmentosa, for example, is a congenital retinal disease affecting the rods. Since the rods are responsible for night vision and vision in dim illumination, a person with Retinitis Pigmentosa will have tunnel vision and night blindness. A rod ERG (performed in dim illumination) on a Retinitis Pigmentosa patient will have a reduced peak.

An example of a cone disorder would be macular degeneration. The cones are responsible for central vision and vision in bright illumination and are located primarily in the macular area of the retina. A person with a macular disorder would have a central field defect and poor acuity. A cone ERG performed on a macular degeneration patient would have a depressed peak.

Color Vision

Human color vision is trichromatic; there are only three types of color pigments in the retina (blue, green and red).

Almost any wavelength of colored light can be matched by a mixture of these three color sensitivities. These three colors are called the primary colors and the sensitivity curves of the primary colors overlap. *(Figure 3-10)*

Every sensation of color can be obtained by some combination of the three primary pigments.

Trichromatic color vision extends to about 30 degrees from the macula. Beyond 30 degrees, the colors red and green become indistinguishable. In the far periphery of the retina, only a few cones exist and all color sense is lost. The peripheral retina has a large number of rods which detect motion but the sensation of color cannot be detected when using peripheral vision.

When a red object is slowly brought into the visual field from the periphery, the observer is first aware of a colorless object. As the red object advances in front, it appears pink or yellow and eventually red.

Our visual acuity is poorest in blue light. This is because we have very few blue cone receptors. In red or green light, our visual sensitivity is much more acute.

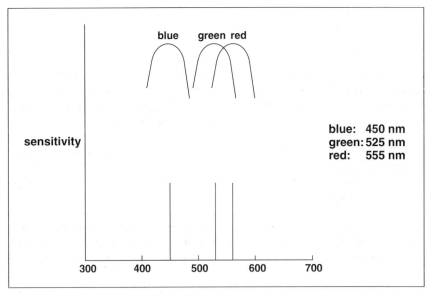

Figure 3-10   Wavelength (nm).

Studies on the rhesus monkey have demonstrated specific color coded cells in the visual area of the brain. These cells are specific for both color and orientation. For example, some brain cells respond to red light oriented horizontally, other cells respond to red light oriented vertically and still other cells respond to red light entering the eye at an angle. The cells appear to be arranged in columns according to color.

An interesting phenomenon of color vision is the afterimage. An afterimage is the complementary of the primary color. When one stares at a red spot for a few minutes and then looks at a white card, a green spot will appear on the card. This is the afterimage. In normal circumstances, this does not cause problems because the eye is continuously moving. A person does not normally stare at an object long enough to form an afterimage.

Complementary colors can also be observed by staring at a grey spot on a red background. The grey spot will eventually appear greenish. Similarly, a grey spot on a green background will eventually appear reddish.

Color Vision Defects

Defective color vision can be either congenital (present at birth) or acquired later in life. Color vision defects are due to an absence of one of the pigments in the photoreceptors. Congenital color defects are either red deficient (called protans), green deficient (called deutans) or blue deficient (called tritans).

Red deficient individuals (protans) lack red pigment in their photoreceptors and are red blind. They cannot identify the color red. Since the sensitivity curve for the red wavelength has minimal overlap with the green and blue sensitivity curves, a red deficient condition is easy to identify.

Green deficient (deutans) and blue deficient individuals (tritans) are more difficult to classify. The sensitivity curves for the visual pigments are more overlapped on the short wavelength side of the peaks. This makes isolation of a blue or green defect more difficult.

Generally, protans and deutans confuse shades of red with shades of green and tritans confuse shades of blue with all other shades. Color deficient individuals confuse shades that normal individuals can easily distinguish.

The genes for red-green defects are sex-linked. In other words, the genes are carried by the female and expressed in the male. A mother carrying the gene for color blindness will pass the defect to half of her male offspring. The probability of a female having a red-green defect is only 0.4%. However, in males there is a 2% chance of a red defect and a 6% chance of a green defect.

Acquired color defects are caused by various diseases or conditions. Certain chemicals, macular disease or optic nerve disease can cause a color vision defect. Blue defects can be caused by Retinitis Pigmentosa or macular disease. Red-green defects can be caused by multiple sclerosis or optic nerve disease. There is a very poor correlation, however, between color vision defects and disease states.

Acquired color vision defects are usually found in only one eye and they frequently vary with time. A congenital vision defect would be present in both eyes and would remain constant through time.

Visual Discrimination

Visual discrimination refers to the ability of the retina to distinguish between certain visual stimuli. The greater the ability to visually discriminate stimuli, the greater the sensitivity. There are three types of visual discrimination: light discrimination, spatial discrimination and temporal discrimination.

Light discrimination refers to brightness sensitivity. It is the ability to detect a very weak light. Light discrimination is the basis for automated visual field testing.

When a patient's visual field is tested, they are instructed to fixate on an object straight ahead while faint lights are flashed in the peripheral field. When the patient notices the flashing light, he is instructed to hit a button which records his response. The light is made dimmer and dimmer until the patient's visual threshold is reached. At this point, the next dimmest light will not be visible to the patient.

Brightness sensitivity is also related to color vision. The greater the illumination, the more true colors will appear. Altering the brightness of an object will affect its color perception. In very poor lighting, discriminating color is impossible since only the rods are stimulated.

Spatial discrimination is the ability to recognize a shape or a pattern such as a letter. It is also the ability to resolve separate parts of the same pattern. CΛT is recognized as the word CAT even though the letter A is not completed. After a pattern has been learned, the brain has the ability to fill in the missing pieces. Spatial discrimination is form recognition.

Temporal discrimination is the ability to detect sensations caused by time varying stimuli such as flickering lights. The classic example is a television set. The lights flicker so fast that it appears as one continuous picture to the human eye. Actually, it is best that we do not have sharp temporal resolution. If our eyes were more discriminating, the television picture would then appear as moving light spots instead of a single image.

Binocular Vision and Stereopsis

Binocular vision is simultaneous vision with two seeing eyes when an object of interest is fixated. The images from both eyes are fused into one; this is called binocular single vision and it is associated with stereopsis. Stereopsis is the binocular perception of depth when two eyes view an object from slightly different vantage points.

Because the two eyes are separated horizontally, the two retinal images are slightly different. This disparity between retinal image sizes provides enough visual information for an estimation of depth. *(Figure 3-11)*

When a person has a sudden loss of vision in one eye, they will experience problems with depth perception. Eventually, monocular cues will

YOUR EYES!

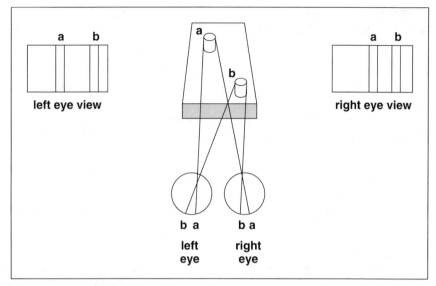

left eye view

right eye view

a

b

b a   b a

left
eye

right
eye

Figure 3-11   Stereopsis.

compensate somewhat although only to a limited extent. The unique perception of stereopsis will be lost, however.

As primates developed during evolution, the eyes moved from a lateral or side position to a frontal position. Binocular vision soon followed this development.

Man's adoption of an upright posture freed the hands and led to the development of manual skills. This led to a further development of hand/eye coordination; the guidance of a binocular visual system controlling the coordinated use of two hands.

Stereoscopic vision improves as an object approaches the eyes. Very distant objects will have very little depth perception.

Try threading a needle with one eye closed and the stereoscopic effect of binocular vision will be greatly appreciated.

Entoptic Phenomena

Entoptic Phenomena are unique visualizations within the eye caused by the structures in the eye. For example, a star does not look like a point of light but as a star because of the lens of the eye which breaks up the rays of light. The visualized star pattern is an entoptic phenomenon.

Another example of an entoptic phenomenon is the visualization of the retinal blood vessels. The blood vessels of the retina lie in front of the photoreceptors and cast a shadow. Under ordinary visual conditions, these vessels are not noticed because the photoreceptors directly under the vessels adapt to the pattern.

When a light is directed into the eye at a certain angle, the shadow of the retinal blood vessels becomes visible. If the light is pressed gently against the outer side of the closed eyelid; the individual can actually see his own blood vessels. The vessels appear as black lace against a red background.

Blue Arcs of the Retina

If a person sits in a dark room facing a red light and fixates slightly to the right of the light, he will notice two bright blue arcs radiating from the light. These are called the blue arcs of the retina. The arcs are horizontal and appear almost immediately. The cause is unknown.

Moore's Lightning Flash

Another interesting visual phenomenon is Moore's lightning flash. It is noticed when first awakening in the morning. The eyes must be moved rapidly from side to side. A bright yellow radiating pattern will appear in each eye. (Figure 3-12) The pattern is called Moore's lightning flash. The image blurs quickly and soon disappears. It is believed to be caused by the vitreous gel moving rapidly over the retina stimulating a light response.

Neurophysiology

The brain and the eye are intimately connected. The optic nerve is actually an extension of the brain. The covering of the brain also extends forward to surround the optic nerve. Furthermore, the orbit of the eye is a passageway to the central nervous system. (The central nervous system consists of the brain and the spinal column). Infections and diseases can pass very easily from the central nervous system to the eye and orbit.

60% of the brain's function involves vision and eye movements. 40% of the axons in the central nervous system pass through the optic chiasm which is part of the visual pathway. Furthermore, eight of the twelve cranial nerves are involved, in some fashion, with vision.

The brain, as it pertains to vision, can be divided into two systems: the afferent system and the efferent system. The afferent system is the sensory

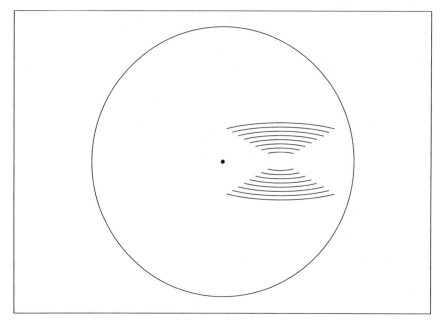

Figure 3-12   Moore's lightning flash.

system, it takes visual information from the retina to the occipital cortex of the brain for processing. The efferent system is the motor system, it acts on the information that is processed in the brain by controlling eye movements and vision.

Duane's Retraction Syndrome

An interesting neurological anomaly is Duane's Retraction Syndrome. The syndrome involves a congenital nerve defect of the sixth cranial nerve, the Abducens Nerve. The sixth nerve is a motor nerve responsible for turning the eye outward. It supplies the lateral rectus muscle.

The syndrome produces a restricted lateral gaze; the eye in question cannot turn outward. When the individual looks to the side of the defect (laterally), the eyelids open wider but the eye movement is restricted. When he looks towards his nose, the eye closes slightly and the eyeball retracts backward.

The condition is not serious and is often misdiagnosed. Patients are often subjected to an extensive neurological evaluation for nothing. Usually, an individual with Duane's Retraction Syndrome will not be aware of the condition. Occasionally, double vision may be experienced on lateral gaze but, in all other directions of gaze, vision will be normal.

Migraine

There are two types of migraine headaches: Classic Migraine and Common Migraine.

Classic Migraine sufferers have a visual aura called a prodrome which precedes the onset of the headache. The prodrome is often a flashing light in the shape of a starlike pattern which slowly expands over a 20 minute period. *(Figure 3-13)* The flashing light pattern is called a scintillating scotoma. This is followed by an intense headache often accompanied by nausea and vomiting.

The migraine patient frequently finds relief by resting in a quiet, dark room until the episode subsides.

A Common Migraine has the same features as a Classic Migraine except the visual aura is not present. The patient experiences the headache without the visual warning.

The typical pattern of a migraine is a follows:

- before age 20: Classic Migraine
- between age 20-40: Common Migraine with nausea
- after the age of 40: headache only

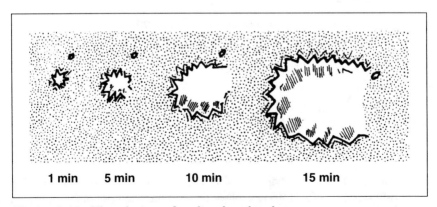

| 1 min | 5 min | 10 min | 15 min |

Figure 3-13 Visual aura of a classic migraine.

Migraines are much more common in females than males. The onset of the migraine frequently occurs at the same time as the onset of menstruation. Pregnancy usually causes the migraine to cease completely or a least reduces its intensity.

There is often a strong family history in migraine sufferers, as high as 70%. Frequently, the patient's mother experienced the same type of headache when she was younger. Individuals who experience car sickness also have a higher incidence of migraine.

The migraine personality is one of a compulsive perfectionist; the so called type A personality. High strung, intense individuals are much more susceptible.

Migraines are caused by a vasoconstriction (narrowing) of the tiny arteries supplying a posterior part of the brain. This results in a reduced oxygen supply through these vessels and apparently triggers an attack. The vasoconstriction of the arteries may be caused by a neuro-electrical response.

Migraine sufferers sometimes find relief by taking aspirin and coffee together. Medications containing ergotamine may abort an attack. Very often, the ergotamine is mixed with caffeine.

Pseudotumor Cerebri (False Tumor of the Brain)

Pseudotumor Cerebri is a neurological disorder caused by increased pressure in the brain; the nerve tissue swells because of increased fluid retention. The condition mimics a brain tumor.

Symptoms include:

- blur outs of vision lasting more than 30 seconds
- transient double vision
- headaches, usually more severe in the morning
- nausea, on occasion

The condition frequently strikes overweight, young females. The individual often had gained a great deal of weight over a short period of time. Premenstrual edema is usually excessive. Birth control pills and hormonal medications have been implicated in Pseudotumor Cerebri.

The patient will have a condition called papilledema which is swelling of the optic nerves due to fluid retention. Indeed, edema of the nerve tissue will be present throughout the central nervous system.

When the eye doctor looks into the back of the eye, he will notice both optic nerves swollen and bulging forward. A visual field analysis will show that both blind spots will be enlarged. This always occurs with papilledema. The blind spot is a normal deficit in the visual field of each eye corresponding to the area of the retina where the optic nerve leaves the back of the eye.

Treatment of the condition consists of diuretics and a restrictive diet limited to about 1,000 calories a day.

Pseudotumor Cerebri is sometimes described as "glaucoma of the brain". Glaucoma results from a build-up of pressure inside the eye. Diuretics are often given for both Pseudotumor Cerebri and glaucoma to help reduce the pressure by eliminating fluid retention.

Pseudotumor Cerebri usually burns out in a few years but in cases where it does not burn out, blindness can result from the sustained high pressure.

Occipital Lobe Disease

The occipital lobe is located in the back of the head. It is the area of the brain where visual information is processed as nerve impulses proceed through the visual pathway. Destruction of the visual cortex will, of course, result in total blindness.

Occipital lobe disease is usually caused by a stroke. A stroke is a sudden restriction of the blood flow to the brain. The vast majority of occipital lobe disorders are vascular in nature; either from hypertension or blocked arteries.

The onset is sudden and often without warning. A visual defect will occur on the opposite side of the constriction. For example, a constriction of the left occipital lobe cortex will cause the right visual field of both eyes to be blacked out.

The episode is caused by a reduced blood flow through arteries supplying the occipital lobe. It usually strikes males in their early 60's. There is frequently a history of diabetes, obesity, smoking or carotid artery disease.

Associated symptoms include the following:

- dizziness
- drop spells
- numbness on both sides of the face, tongue and mouth

YOUR EYES!

Any of these symptoms should be investigated promptly since there is a good chance that a stroke has taken place.

4

Refractive Errors and
Their Correction

Good Vision is More Than 20/20

20/20 does not mean perfect vision. It simply means that you have normal clear vision at a 20 foot distance. Effective vision requires many other skills, such as eye alignment and focusing ability. 20/20 vision means that at 20 feet, a person sees the size letter on the examination chart that most people without a refractive error see at 20 feet. If at this 20 foot distance, a person cannot read letters smaller than those normally read at a distance of 40 feet, then he has 20/40 vision. The larger the bottom number of the fraction, the more blurred the vision.

Another way to look at visual acuity is, if a person has 20/40 vision, they can see no better than the 40 foot line of the chart at 20 feet away. Someone with 20/20 vision can see the 40 foot line of the chart clearly at 40 feet away. Some people have better than 20/20 vision, say 20/15. This means the person can see the 15 foot line of the chart when standing 20 feet away. Someone with 20/20 vision would have to be standing 15 feet away from the chart in order to see that line.

When someone has 20/20 vision, it does not necessarily mean he has normal vision at closer distances. At nearer distances, his vision may be blurred. It is important to have clear vision at all distances, such as for reading, not just 20 feet and beyond. It is also important to achieve this good vision rapidly because you are constantly changing focus from distance to near and back again. Your eyes must also be able to follow an object and point quickly and accurately from one object to another. Both eyes must work together as a team and be able to converge rapidly or point to an object simultaneously as it moves.

You must also have good peripheral (side vision) awareness and be able to judge the distance or position of things. You must also be able to interpret what is seen with speed and efficiency.

You can see, therefore, that 20/20 measures only one aspect of vision, namely visual acuity. Clear, comfortable, efficient vision involves much more.

Common Refractive Errors

Hyperopia or Farsightedness

Farsightedness is a type of vision in which seeing is clearer at far distances than at near. *(Figures 4-1 and 4-2)* When the eye is relaxed, the combined powers of its optical elements is not enough to bring things into focus. The

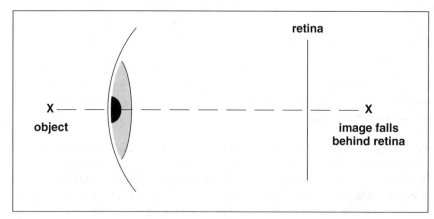

Figure 4-1 Farsightedness – image of an object falls behind the retina and is thus, out of focus.

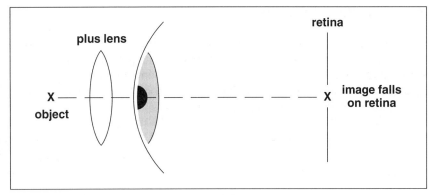

Figure 4-2 **Plus lens in front of eye (either glasses or contacts) increases the focusing ability of the eye and brings the image forward, focusing on the retina. This results in clear vision.**

person who is farsighted must maintain a focusing effort to keep things clear when focusing at a distance and an even greater effort to keep things focused at near. This focusing effort frequently causes fatigue and discomfort.

Do not assume that farsightedness simply means clear distance vision and blurred near vision. If a person has good focusing ability or just a little hyperopia, he may be able to maintain both clear distance and clear near vision. If, on the other hand, a person has poor focusing ability or a high amount of hyperopia, he cannot focus efficiently even for far vision. This person's vision will be blurred for both distance and near, although greater for near.

Symptoms of farsightedness include difficulty in maintaining clear vision in reading, difficulty concentrating and fatigue after close work. Headaches with close work, tension, burning eyes and extending the reading material away from the eyes may also develop. Other symptoms can include nervousness after sustained visual concentration, irritability and even nausea.

The solution to farsightedness is either glasses or contact lenses. The lenses supply the needed focus that the eyes are lacking. This reduces the focusing effort and results in clear, comfortable vision. In farsightedness, the image of an object falls behind the retina and is, thus, out of focus. Plus lenses are used to correct farsightedness. A plus lens is thicker in the middle than on the edge. It brings the image of an object forward, focusing on the retina, resulting in clear vision.

YOUR EYES!

Myopia or Nearsightedness

Nearsightedness is a type of vision in which seeing is clearer at close distances than at far. *(Figures 4-3 and 4-4)* With nearsightedness, there is always some blur at distance and there is always some point at near that will be clear. If a person is very nearsighted, the near point of clear vision can be very close, up to two or three inches from the eye.

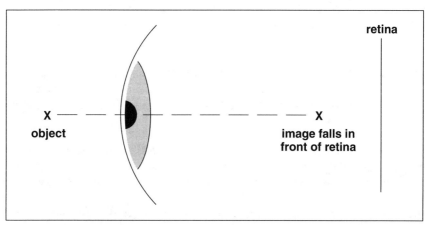

Figure 4-3 Nearsightedness – image of an object falls in front of retina and is thus, out of focus.

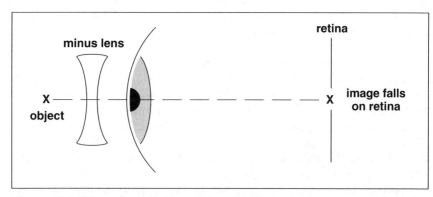

Figure 4-4 Minus lens in front of eye (either glasses or contacts) decreases the focusing ability of the eye and brings the image backward, focusing on the retina. This results in clear vision.

Nearsightedness usually begins to develop during the teen years. It is usually not present in early childhood. Generally, myopia gets worse during its early stages and can progress rapidly during adolescence. It stabilizes during the early adult years. It often decreases during the middle adult years and can increase again in late adulthood.

Many times people are not aware that their distance vision is becoming blurry because of the gradual onset of myopia. Nearsighted individuals with vision as poor as 20/200 sometimes are not aware that their vision is failing. This is one reason that vision exams should be performed on a regular basis.

Simple myopia usually does not cause discomfort since the eye does not have to make any adaptation as with farsightedness. In nearsightedness, the image of an object falls in front of the retina and is, thus, out of focus. The remedy is either eyeglasses or contact lenses. Minus lenses are used to correct nearsightedness. A minus lens is thicker on the edge than in the middle. It moves the image of an object backward, focusing on the retina, resulting in clear vision.

Astigmatism

As defined by Webster, "astigmatism is a structural defect of the eye that prevents light rays from an object from meeting in a single focal point, so that indistinct images are formed." *(Figure 4-5)*

By holding a magnifying glass in the sun, the rays of sunlight can be brought into a sharp focus. Now if that same magnifying glass were elastic and could be squeezed from opposite sides and became oblong instead of round, the image would not come to a point. The surface of the magnifying glass would be astigmatic and this would result in a blurred image.

Most astigmatism takes place on the cornea, the front surface of the eye. A non-astigmatic cornea would be similar to the round magnifying glass, which would have no effect on the incoming light rays. The rays would focus to a point on the retina. With an astigmatic eye, the cornea is not spherical and the light rays cannot focus to a point.

Another way to think of astigmatism is to compare the shape of a basketball with a football. A basketball has the same shape in all directions and a football is curved more in one direction than in the other. An astigmatic cornea would be shaped more like a football than a basketball. The difference in curves results in distortion and a blurred image.

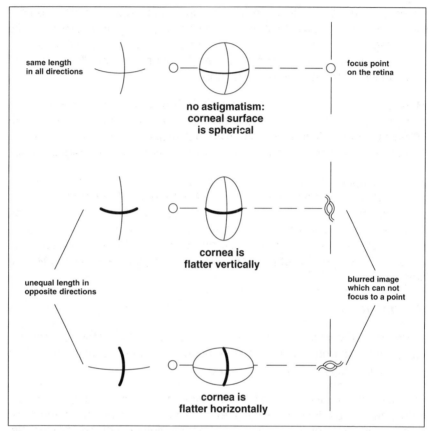

same length
in all directions

focus point
on the retina

no astigmatism:
corneal surface
is spherical

unequal length in
opposite directions

cornea is
flatter vertically

blurred image
which can not
focus to a point

cornea is
flatter horizontally

Figure 4-5 Astigmatism.

Astigmatism is the most common refractive error, occurring to some degree in about 90% of all eyes. Small amounts cause very little distortion but may cause headaches or fatigue. When astigmatism is corrected by glasses or contact lenses, things often look distorted or slanted for awhile until the wearer adapts. Astigmatism can occur in combination with either far-sightedness or nearsightedness.

Amblyopia

Amblyopia means unexplained reduction in clearness of vision. Sometimes it is incorrectly called "lazy eye." Even with proper corrective lenses and no detectable eye disease, the vision is still below normal. Amblyopia usually involves just one eye. Only central vision is affected, leaving the side vision intact.

The exact cause of amblyopia is unknown. It develops almost exclusively in persons with an eyeturn or a large difference in refractive errors between the two eyes.

Since amblyopia occurs in one eye only, children are usually not aware of it. And it is generally more treatable at an early age. A pediatric evaluation should, therefore, include an evaluation for amblyopia. Remedies include patching of the better eye, forcing the amblyopic eye to work and training techniques that teach the eye to function properly.

Presbyopia

As a person ages, he loses the ability to focus clearly at the reading distance. This is presbyopia. The age at which this occurs varies but is generally between 40 and 50. Presbyopia is a gradual loss of focusing ability and is normal for everyone. It is not a disease.

The signs of presbyopia include blurred vision at the reading distance and a need to hold reading material further away. Other symptoms include headache, fatigue or difficulty concentrating when doing close work.

Presbyopia is not preventable but can be compensated for with contact lenses or eyeglasses – either bifocal or multifocal lenses or reading glasses. Bifocals or multifocals are needed if there is a distance correction that must also be compensated for in one pair of glasses. As the focusing ability of the eyes is reduced gradually over time, the near correction must be made stronger periodically.

When prescribing a correction for presbyopia, it is important to determine the distance the patient will be holding the material when wearing the correction. Different working distances require different corrections. Holding material at 13 inches requires a stronger correction than at 20 inches.

Focusing Difficulty

In addition to focusing sharply at the reading distance, it must also be done quickly and easily. If not, comfortable near vision cannot be achieved. Glasses for near work may be needed to reduce fatigue and discomfort. If focusing is slow and difficult, reading will be slow and difficult.

Eye Teaming Difficulty

Good vision also includes the ability of both eyes to aim at the same object simultaneously. This should be automatic and smooth. Both eyes must work at a team. If not, double vision will be present or the brain blocks out the image of one eye. Most cases of poor eye coordination are the result of improper muscle control. Each eye has six extraocular muscles and they all must be functioning as a team or improper alignment results.

Double vision (diplopia) from faulty alignment is very uncomfortable and the brain tends to suppress one image to restore visual comfort. Sometimes an extra muscular effort is required to maintain alignment and this frequently causes headache, fatigue and general discomfort. The ability of the eyes to work together is also necessary for good depth perception.

Remedies include correcting any refractive error which is present and visual training to re-educate youngsters with eye coordination problems. Prisms are sometimes used to correct eye coordination difficulties. A prism is a lens that does not change the focusing of the light but rather its direction. A prism changes the direction of the light entering the eyes so that a similar image falls on corresponding parts of the back of both eyes. This compensates for the eye misalignment; the eyes will see as if they are pointing in the same direction.

Strabismus

The condition in which the eyes are not properly aligned with each other is called strabismus. It is sometimes called a squint or a tropia. The usual cause is faulty muscle control or a failure to learn to use both eyes as a team. Only one eye crosses, the other points to the object being seen. An eye can turn either in or out, up or down.

Anisometropia

This is a condition of the eyes in which they have unequal refractive power (unequal amounts of farsightedness, nearsightedness or astigmatism). One eye will be in focus and the other one will not. The out of focus eye, if untreated, can become amblyopic. Proper correction is important to allow the brain to fuse two clear images instead of one clear image and one blurry one.

Radial Keratotomy

Eighty percent of the refractive power of the eye comes from the front part of the cornea. Modifying the front curve of the cornea is the basis for surgery that corrects refractive disorders.

The most common type of refractive surgery is radial keratotomy. *(Figure 4-6)* So far, over 100,000 radial keratotomy procedures have been performed in this country. The surgery was perfected by Dr. Fyodorov of the Soviet Union and was introduced to this country in 1980.

Radial keratotomy improves myopia (nearsightedness) by surgically flattening the outer part of the cornea. Eight radial incisions of equal depth are made in the cornea. Sometimes, four or sixteen incisions are made, but

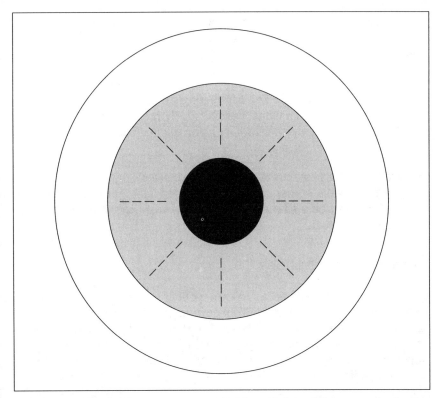

Figure 4-6 Radial keratotomy – eight radial incisions made in the cornea.

generally eight incisions will give the expected result. Most procedures are done with just a topical anesthetic, but it is very important that any eye movements during the surgery be restricted.

What type of results can be expected with this type of surgery? As with any type of refractive surgery, 20/20 vision is not always achieved. Overpromoting radial keratotomy as a way of eliminating eyeglasses will result in many dissatisfied patients. The procedure is not for everyone. Generally, for moderate amounts of nearsightedness, good results can be expected.

In 1985, the National Eye Institute published results of a five year study called the *Perspective Evaluation of Radial Keratotomy* or *PERK*. With low myopia, vision was improved to 20/40 or better in 92% of patients. For patients with moderate amounts of myopia, 20/40 or better was obtained in 81% of the cases. As for highly myopic patients, 20/40 or better vision was achieved in 63% of the cases. Remember, the procedure does not guarantee everyone will see 20/20 afterwards without glasses or contacts, but generally vision will be improved.

Major complications from the surgery are rare but there are some minor problems which can occur. These include glare, awareness of a sunburst pattern, astigmatism, infections, vessel growth through the cornea and farsightedness. Sometimes there is fluctuating vision, poor night vision and the inability to wear contact lenses if needed.

Despite these possible complications, radial keratotomy is a safe and reasonably predictable surgery with generally satisfactory results. Like any type of elective surgery, it is not for everyone. And the long term results have yet to be determined.

Eyeglass Prescriptions

It is important for the eye doctor to know your current eyeglass prescription when he does the examination. Your current prescription can be read from your old pair of eyeglasses or obtained from the records of your previous examination. A device called a lensometer is used to read the prescription from the eyeglasses. By law, you are entitled to your prescription and it can usually be obtained over the telephone.

By assessing your current prescription, the examining doctor can tell if there is a big change in your refractive error and can prescribe accordingly.

Sometimes it is prudent not to prescribe a big change in the eyeglass prescription; the patient will have difficulty adapting. As a rule, the older the patient the more difficult it is to adapt to the new prescription. Children can accept big changes in their eyeglass correction while senior citizens cannot.

Another good reason to bring your current pair of eyeglasses or the written prescription when being examined is the possible detection of eye disease. The classic example is diabetes. Frequent changes in the eyeglass prescription can be an indication of early, undetected diabetes. Very often the optometrist is the first one to suspect diabetes based solely on the eye examination.

Corneal disease, cataracts and macular disease can also cause changes in the refractive error. Corneal disease and age-related cataracts often result in an increase in nearsightedness. Macular edema can result in an increase in farsightedness since the edema forces the retina forward and the focusing point, thus, further behind the retina.

Eyeglasses

There are five basic face shapes: round, oval, heart, rectangular and square. Generally, you should not wear a particular shaped frame on the same shaped face. A round shaped frame, for example, will not look that well on a person with a round face. A rectangular or squared off frame will look better. People with heart shaped faces are the most difficult to fit with eyeglasses. They will do best by staying away from pilot or goggle-shaped glasses.

People with long, rectangular faces should not wear temples coming off the top part of the frame. This makes the face appear too long. Short faces look better with the temples coming off the top of the frame. This gives the face a longer appearance.

The oval-shaped face is the easiest to fit; people with this shape can wear just about any shape in eyeglasses. People without oval faces should determine their face shape and select eyewear with a different shape.

Selection of frame color is often difficult. As a rule, the lighter the hair color, the lighter the frame. Dark haired individuals look better in dark frames.

Another system involves using skin tones, eye color and hair color to determine if a person is a warm tone or a cool tone. Patients are separated into cool colors (summer or winter) or warm colors (autumn or spring). People in

YOUR EYES!

the cool category have white skin and blonde hair without red undertones or dark hair with olive or dark skin. People in the warm category have pale skin, strawberry blonde, red or light brown hair and red skin tones.

A "cool" person looks good in blue or grey frames and a "warm" person looks best in brown frames. A "cool" person looks best in pink tints and a "warm" person looks best in tan tints.

There are two general types of lenses for eyeglasses: plastic and glass. Plastic is lighter and more comfortable but scratches easier. Glass is heavier but is much more difficult to scratch. A special type of plastic called polycarbonate is the closest thing to unbreakable but is also easy to scratch. Safety lenses, which must be able to withstand great impact, are made of polycarbonate. Lenses in sport frames, such as for racquetball, are also polycarbonate. Also, if a patient has only one functioning eye, it is a good idea for this patient to wear polycarbonate lenses. It would be very unfortunate to have an injury to the healthy eye, rendering the patient totally blind. With regular plastic lenses and in particular glass lenses, the odds of an eye injury from a shattered lens are much greater than with polycarbonate lenses.

With very high prescriptions, polycarbonate lenses are thinner and more cosmetically flattering than standard plastic lenses. Polycarbonate lenses are coated at the lab with a scratch resistant coating. Regular plastic lenses can also be coated at the patient's request.

Photochromatic lenses, which become darker in bright sunlight and lighten indoors, must be glass.

Glass lenses generally cannot be placed in rimless frames and not all prescriptions can be placed in all frames. If a person has a high prescription, (and thus will have thick lenses), they must select frames that are not too large. The bigger the eyesize of the frame, the thicker the lenses. People with very high prescriptions are somewhat limited in their frame selection.

Somewhere on the frame there will be the following information:

- Eye size
- Bridge size
  - The eye and bridge size are written 54/20, for example.
- Temple length

– The temple length is listed separately: 140, for example.

- Color
  – The color is either listed as a color or a number code, usually 3 or 4 numbers.
- Manufacturer
- Name of frame
  – The manufacturer's name is usually imprinted somewhere and the frame's particular name will also be listed.

If you are copying information from a frame, you will need all of the above information if you plan on purchasing it elsewhere.

Bifocal Types and other Multifocals

Different multifocals are better suited for different needs. *(Figure 4-7)* Listed below are the more common types of multifocals. Bifocals allow near and distance vision but no intermediate vision. Trifocals allow near, intermediate and distance vision. Progressives give near, intermediate and distance vision and everything in between. For most people, near vision is at 16 inches, intermediate vision is about 22 inches and distance vision is 2 feet and beyond.

The most common type of multifocal is the flat top 25 bifocal. It is an excellent all purpose lens. The executive bifocal is ideal for sitting and doing prolonged near work such as accounting. It is not a good choice for everyday wear since steps and curbs are difficult to notice when wearing an executive. Walking up and down stairs can be particularly hazardous.

Trifocals are fine for computer use and other intermediate range tasks but people often have a difficult time adapting to them.

The great breakthrough in ophthalmic lenses in the past few years has been the progressive. There are no visible lines and, unlike the other multifocals, all ranges of vision can be brought into focus. The progressive lens is the most remarkable correction today for presbyopia. It comes closer than any other multifocal in simulating the human eye's focusing ability. With a slight head tilt up or down, the correct focusing position can be found. The progressive has an infinite number of focusing positions from distance to near, not just distance, intermediate and near. *(Figure 4-8)*

YOUR EYES!

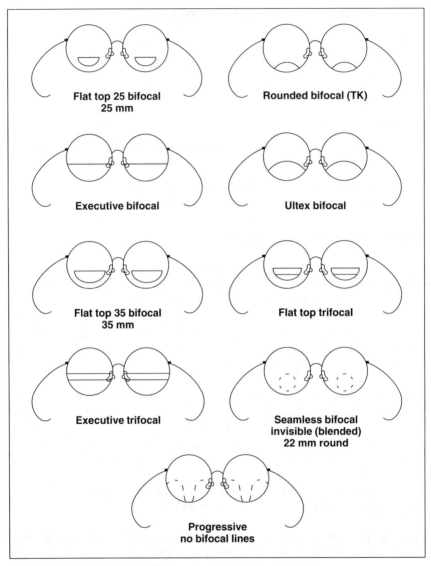

Figure 4-7 The different types of multifocal lenses.

One drawback to the progressive is a period of adaptation lasting from a few days to a few weeks. However, most people adapt very nicely. The key to using a progressive successfully is simply to point your nose at wherever

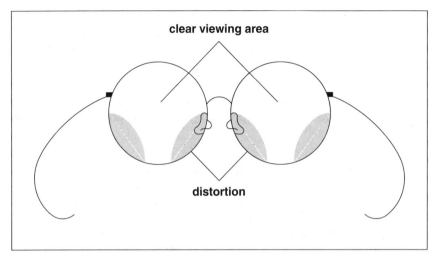

clear viewing area

distortion

Figure 4-8 Progressive.

you are looking. You cannot move your eyes laterally; you must move your head and point your nose at your viewing target. After a short period, the brain will pick up on this and do it automatically. The peripheral part of the progressive lens has distortion and moving only your eyes and not your head results in viewing through this distorted area.

Lens Coatings

There are three basic types of lens coatings which can be applied to eyeglass lenses: a scratch resistant coating, an anti-reflective coating and an ultraviolet filter (coating).

Scratch resistant coatings are used on plastic and polycarbonate lenses only. The scratch resistant coating is usually applied by the manufacturer, although it can be done at the laboratory. The coating will not increase the scratch resistance of glass lenses. Glass lenses, however, need no scratch coating. They are the ultimate in scratch resistant lenses. The disadvantage of glass lenses is, of course, the weight. Glass lenses are about twice as heavy as plastic lenses.

An anti-reflective coating is actually a series of coatings applied to the lens at the laboratory. Originally, the anti-reflective coating was a single layer coating, but it did not work well on all parts of the spectrum.

Anti-reflective coatings work by increasing the amount of light transmitted through the lens. Light is transmitted almost 100%. Increasing the transmission of light reduces the amount of reflection. To optimally reduce all of the reflection, the laboratory uses several layers of coating each having a slightly different thickness. This is called a broad band coating and it allows transmission of almost all of the light over the entire spectrum.

With anti-reflective coatings, annoying reflections virtually disappear. There is a marked improvement in vision for most wearers, particularly at night. Ghost images are eliminated.

People with high prescriptions (thick lenses) do well with an anti-reflective coating; improving the cosmetics of the lenses as well as their vision. The main disadvantage of anti-reflective lenses is that they are difficult to keep clean. When they become dirty, it reduces their effectiveness. They are also somewhat expensive and the laboratory often takes an extra week for processing. However, aside from these disadvantages, an anti-reflective coating is probably the best add on feature available for lenses today improving both the cosmetic appearance of the lenses and the patient's vision.

An ultraviolet coating is a clear dye applied to the lens. This blocks the transmission of ultraviolet light which can be harmful to the eye. Ultraviolet radiation (primarily from the sun) has been implicated in cataract formation and certain retinal disorders such as macular degeneration. Patients who have had cataracts removed must wear eyewear with ultraviolet protection. The lens of the eye is the main absorber of ultraviolet light. The lens shields the harmful rays from the retina. When the lens of the eye is removed (cataract surgery), the retina is directly exposed to ultraviolet radiation.

Most cataract surgeons opt for an intraocular implant which replaces the patient's old lens. Many of these implants nowadays have ultraviolet protection built into them. It is still a good idea, however, for these patients to wear eyewear with ultraviolet protection.

People who work outdoors should also wear ultraviolet lenses. As a rule, an ultraviolet coating (filter) is a good idea for everyone since we are all susceptible to ultraviolet radiation. There are no disadvantages to wearing glasses with ultraviolet protection. The coating is inexpensive, has no effect on the optics of the lens and is warranted for the life of the lens. When an ultraviolet coating is applied, it cannot be removed and does not lose its effectiveness over time.

Photochromatics

A photochromatic lens is a glass lens that changes from very dark in sunlight to almost clear indoors. They are only available in glass.

There are four types of photochromatics available today. They are photogray extra, photobrown extra, photosun II and photogray II.

Photogray extra is a fast acting, all purpose lens that works well under most lighting conditions. When indoors and fully faded it transmits 85% of visible light, leaving just a residual tint. When in bright sunlight, it blocks out about 80% of the light comparing favorably with a dark, fixed tint pair of sunglasses. It takes about one minute to darken into sunglasses and it takes about five minutes indoors to become clear again. It also offers excellent ultraviolet and anti-glare protection.

Photobrown extra has properties similar to photogray extra. Photobrown extra looks better cosmetically and is generally more popular with women. On hazy days, it appears to give better vision. As with photogray extra, it is also excellent for ultraviolet protection.

The photosun II is the darkest photchromatic available. Unlike the other photochromatics, it becomes lighter as the sunlight diminishes in strength. When fully faded, it transmits only 40% of the visible light making it ideal for a cloudy day. It is generally too dark for indoor use and cannot be worn for night driving. It is, however, an excellent lens for very bright sunlight and outdoor sports.

Photogray II is the fastest acting of the photochromatics, darkening outdoors in about one minute. In its faded state, it is the clearest of the photochromatics transmitting about 87% of the visible light. In its darkened state, it blocks about 60% of the light, making it a comfortable pair of sunglasses. It is not quite strong enough for very bright sunlight or prolonged activity outdoors on very sunny days. It is considered a medium shade sunglass.

Anti-reflective coatings can be applied to all photchromatic lenses. The coatings will increase light transmittance by about 7%. All bifocals and progressive lenses can be ordered in photogray extra or photobrown extra.

In short, photochromatics are an excellent option when considering sunglasses. You only need one pair of glasses for both outdoors and indoors (with the exception of photosun II which is strictly for outdoors). The photochromatics offer excellent ultraviolet protection and anti-reflective coatings can be applied to the lenses. The only drawback is that glass lenses are somewhat heavy.

Polarizing Lenses

Any lens that reduces unwanted glare or annoying light results in more comfortable vision. Light bouncing off a non-shiny surface is not irritating but light reflected off a shiny surface can be quite annoying.

Reflected glare consists of polarized rays; light that is confined to one direction. The incoming light is at right angles to the line of vision. Polarized lenses consist of thin plastic sheets stretched to give an elliptical shape. The plastic sheet allows transmission of light in one direction and blocks it completely 90 degrees away.

Polarized lenses can be either glass or plastic, with a laminating piece of thin plastic stretched between two lens components.

Polarizing lenses are ideal for anyone exposed to a water surface; fisherman, lifeguards, boaters, etc. It is much easier viewing through the surface of the water with polarized lenses. People who drive a lot also benefit from polarization since it reduces glare from highway surfaces. In addition, any sunglass shade can be made in polarized lenses.

Wearing polarized lenses allows colors to be more true by reducing the scattering of white light. Reds will be redder, blues will be bluer. It allows for more comfortable, natural vision. Furthermore, all ultraviolet radiation will be blocked with polarized lenses.

Polarized lenses are available in both single vision and bifocal corrections. The only major drawback is the price; polarized prescription lenses can be quite expensive. But for people who are very sensitive to outdoor glare, nothing works as well as polarization.

Fashion Tints

With glass lenses, the coloring process is through the entire lens. With plastic lenses, a tint is applied to the outside of the lens. People with high prescriptions must be careful when ordering tinted glass lenses. The thicker the lens, the darker the glass. Also, the coloring will not appear even throughout the lens. The thicker part of the lens (the edge in minus prescriptions and the center in plus prescriptions) will be darker.

Plastic lenses that are tinted will appear more even and there is a greater variety of tints available. The entire lens can be tinted or the top can be tinted and the bottom left clear (gradient tint). It is even possible with plastic lenses to have one shade at the top and a different shade at the bottom.

Light tints (10 to 30%) afford glare protection; particularly from overhead fluorescent lights and also from video display terminals. Gradient tints are ideal for overhead glare reduction.

Tints that are very dark can exaggerate shadows and lines around the eyes. Yellow and green tints are not especially flattering. Most people look good in pinks and blues. Pink and flesh tones help hide lines around the eyes. Tints can also improve the appearance of high prescriptions by reducing the magnification look of plus lenses and the edge thickness of minus lenses.

Contact Lenses

Leonardo da Vinci, in 1508, was the first person to describe contact lenses for the correction of a refractive error. His concept of neutralizing the refractive error of the cornea is the basis of the contact lens. One suggestion of his was to place a small half sphere filled with water over the eye to correct the refractive error.

In 1636, René Descartes was the first person to suggest placing a lens directly onto the cornea but it was not until 1887 that the first contact lens with refractive power was actually developed. In 1888, A. Eugen Fick placed a spherical glass spectacle directly on the cornea and this is considered the first true corneal contact lens.

The first American to develop synthetic plastics for contact lenses was William Feinbloom. The plastic was lighter than glass and much easier to shape. In 1936, the Rohm and Haas company developed the transparent plastic methyl methacrylate which is used frequently today. In 1955, George Butterfield recognized that the shape of the contact lens should approximate the shape of the cornea. This principle is used in fitting the majority of contact lenses today.

Many others contributed, both here and abroad, to the development of contact lenses as we know them today, with many individuals working independently toward similar solutions.

There are over 18 million contact lens wearers in the United States today. About 2.5 million wear hard contacts, 2.5 million wear gas permeable contacts, over 9 million wear soft daily wear contacts and over 4 million wear soft extended wear contacts. Over 65% of all contact lens wearers are female and over half are between the ages of 25 and 44 (from an 1989 FDA survey).

Hard Spherical Corneal Contacts and Gas Permeable Contact Lenses

These lenses are fit smaller than the iris and larger than the pupil when dilated. The anterior and posterior sides are both spherical. These lenses are used to correct myopia, hyperopia and astigmatism.

Hard or rigid contact lenses are made of polymethylmethacrylate (PMMA). It is the most durable material available. It is not, however, gas permeable as the material is nonporous. The initial rigid lenses were all PMMA. Despite their durability, PMMA lenses have no flexibility and will chip or break if excess pressure is applied to the lens. PMMA lenses must move freely on the eye to permit oxygen to reach the cornea through tear exchange. Nowadays, however, most rigid lenses dispensed are gas permeable materials.

Gas permeable lenses are made from newer, porous materials such as silicone. They also move freely on the eye to allow oxygen to reach the cornea through the tears; however, oxygen can also be exchanged through the lens material itself. Because of this added permeability, gas permeable rigid lenses are much healthier than the old PMMA hard contacts. They may not last as long, but gas permeable lenses are definitely the rigid lens of choice.

Advantages of Hard (PMMA) Contact Lenses:

- longest life span of all contact lenses
- excellent vision
- the least expensive
- easiest to clean

Disadvantages of Hard (PMMA) Contact Lenses:

- gradual build-up of wearing time required
- lenses uncomfortable during breaking-in period
- lenses are easily dislodged
- corneal edema develops more readily
- vision is blurred when switching back and forth from contacts to glasses

Advantages of Gas Permeable Contact Lenses:

- oxygen flows through lens material resulting in a healthier cornea
- generally, more comfortable than PMMA lenses
- excellent vision
- no corneal edema
- no blurred vision when switching back and forth from glasses to contacts

Disadvantages of Gas Permeable Contact Lenses:

- gradual build-up of wearing time required
- lenses uncomfortable during breaking-in period
- lenses are easily dislodged
- oil and protein deposits on the lens develop quicker than PMMA lenses

Parameters of Rigid Lenses

PMMA and gas permeable contacts are generally more difficult to fit and require more time with the doctor. Unlike soft contacts, rigid lenses must be fit exactly to the shape of the cornea. *(Figure 4-9)* In a sense, they are custom made. The doctor must consider the following parameters when fitting and ordering rigid contacts:

- power of the lens (canceling out the patient's refractive error)
- diameter of the lens
- base curve of the lens or central posterior curve (the primary curve of the concave side of the lens designed to fit the anterior surface of the cornea)
- optic zone (the diameter of the posterior central curve)
- the intermediate and peripheral curves of the lens
- the thickness of the lens
- the blend of the peripheral curves
- the edge bevel (how the lens is tapered)
- the color
- type of material

The Care and Handling of Rigid Lenses

Before the lenses are handled, the hands should be washed, preferably with a soap that does not contain creams. Creamy soaps leave a residue on the fingers which can put a film on the lenses. Eye make-up must be removed before retiring and the outer eye area should be cleansed thoroughly, especially if oils are used to remove make-up. Oils and creams remaining on the lids and lashes can easily find their way into the tears and then onto the lenses.

Insertion of Rigid Lenses:

- After washing your hands, handle the lenses over a table with a mirror placed flat on the surface.

- The lens is placed on the tip of the index finger. Bend over and face the mirror. Use the other arm to reach over your head and place the middle finger firmly over the upper lid. Lift the upper lid with this finger.

- The middle finger of the hand with the lens is used to pull down the lower lid.

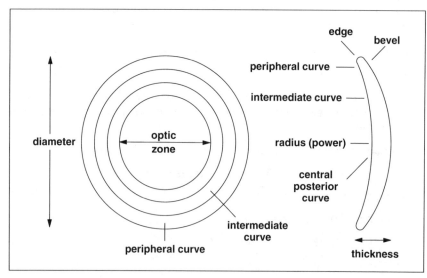

Figure 4-9 Rigid contact lens.

- Looking straight ahead into the mirror, the lens is placed directly onto the cornea.

- When the lens is in place, look down and release the lids.

Removal of Rigid Lenses:

- Again, the hands are washed.

- Bend over a mirror which is lying flat on a table.

- Look directly into the mirror. For removing the right lens, the head is tilted slightly to the right. With left lens removal, the head is tilted slightly to the left.

- The eyes are then opened as wide as possible.

- The index finger is placed at the outer corner of the eye. With the index finger, pull tightly out and upward and blink lens out of the eye.

Another Method of Lens Removal:

Check to make sure that the contact lens is positioned between the lids. Place index finger over lower lid and press gently. With the other index finger, press in and down on the upper lid forcing the lens to tip out of the eye. By holding the lower lid firmly, the lens cannot slide under the lower lid when pressure is applied from above. The lens hits the lower lid and tips outward.

When wearing rigid lenses, they can sometimes move off center causing the new patient to panic. The lens, however, cannot go behind the eye. If it gets stuck behind the upper lid and cannot be found, it will usually find its way back to the front part of the eye again. If it stays lodged under the upper lid, an eye doctor can evert the lid and remove the lens. If the lens is off center and visible, it is easy for the patient to re-center it without removing it. The edge of the lens farthest from the cornea should be gently pressed and the lens is then slowly slid back onto the cornea.

Rigid contact lens wearers must learn proper blinking techniques. This is important to insure proper tear exchange under the lens and to help reduce lens awareness. Blinking exercises include looking upward and blinking several times slowly and deliberately. Also, looking to the extreme right and left and blinking repeatedly. Eventually, proper blinking will become a natural part of lens wear and the patient will not have to be consciously aware of it.

First time rigid contact lens wearers must realize that the adaptation period for the first few weeks can be very trying. Symptoms include lens awareness, blurred vision, tearing, sensitivity to light and tired eyes. Assuming the fit is correct (the doctor's responsibility), the symptoms should gradually diminish resulting in comfortable wear. Sometimes, even if the fit is correct, the patient just cannot tolerate rigid lenses and other alternatives must be pursued.

The wearing schedule for rigid lenses is determined by the doctor but the usual schedule is as follows:

- Day 1: 3 hours
- Day 2: 4 hours
- Day 3: 5 hours
- Day 4: 6 hours
- Day 5: 7 hours
- Day 6: 8 hours
- Day 7: should be a follow-up visit with the doctor to determine how well the patient is adapting to the new lenses. If everything is fine, the wearing schedule is gradually increased further to a maximum of all waking hours. It should be noted, however, that not all patients can wear contact lenses for all waking hours. It is also important to realize that speeding up the wearing schedule offers no advantage and may actually compromise the eye.

First time contact lens wearers must be aware of a few other points. They cannot rub their eyes or sleep or swim with their lenses on. They should not switch solutions unless consulting with their doctor first and, if a foreign body gets under the lens, the lens should be removed and cleaned before reinsertion. The lens should not be over-worn and they must return in one week for their progress evaluation and all other follow-up care. If they have any questions, they should not hesitate to call their practitioner.

Soft Contact Lenses

Soft contact lenses are fit larger that the iris and are used to correct hyperopia, myopia and astigmatism. They are made from soft, pliable materials which allow oxygen to pass through the lens. Soft contacts adhere to the cornea and move vary slightly with the blink.

Advantages of Soft Contact Lenses:

- the adaptation period is minimal, often just a few hours
- the lenses can be worn inconsistently
- generally, foreign bodies do not get trapped under the lens
- the lenses are not easily dislodged
- the comfort is generally much better than rigid lenses

Disadvantages of Soft Contact Lenses:

- vision is not as sharp as rigid lenses
- lenses are not as durable as rigid lenses
- cleaning procedures are more involved than with rigid lenses
- lens dehydration can result in reduced comfort and blurred vision
- increased chance of eye infections
- oil and protein deposits from the tears form easily on the lenses

The Care and Handling of Soft Lenses

The hands should be washed before the lenses are inserted. The lenses are then rinsed with saline. Care must be taken when handling soft contacts since they are fragile. New soft contact lens wearers frequently tear a lens while cleaning it or when removing it from the case or the eye.

Insertion of Soft Contact Lenses (Figure 4-10)

- the lens is placed on the tip of the index finger. Check to make sure that it is not inside out. The proper position is rounded with the edges pointed inward. An inside out lens has the edges pointing outward giving the lens a bowl shaped appearance. An inside out lens may be uncomfortable and blur the vision.
- look directly into a mirror. Use the other arm to reach over your head and place the middle finger firmly over the upper lid.
- lift the upper lid with this finger.
- the middle finger of the hand with the lens is used to pull down the lower lid.
- place the lens directly onto the cornea while watching your eye in the mirror.

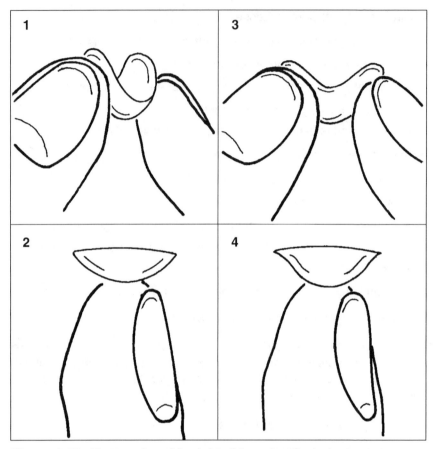

**Figure 4-10 Figures 1 and 2: right side out soft contact.
Figures 3 and 4: inside out soft contact.**

- without releasing the lids, move the lens around until the air bubbles are released.
- look downward and slowly releases the lids.

Removal of Soft Contact Lenses

- look up slightly.
- the middle finger pulls down the lower lid.
- the index finger of the same hand is placed on the lens, and the lens is then slid downward onto the white part of the eye (sclera).

- without removing your index finger from the lens, place your thumb on the lens and pinch the lens gently, releasing the suction which holds the lens in place.
- squeeze the lens between your thumb and index finger and slowly pull it away.

When you are not sure if the lens is in place, cover the other eye and see if the vision is clear. If the vision is good, the lens must be centered on the cornea. Do not poke at the cornea if the lens is not there. Sometimes, people assume that the lens is on the cornea when it is not and attempt to slide the lens down and grab it. This can result in a corneal abrasion. Also, the lenses should not be removed if they are dehydrated. Often after sleeping with the lenses, they become dried out and do not move freely on the eye. Do not try to remove these lenses until after comfort drops are used to rehydrate them. Sometimes, drops have to be applied for several minutes before the lenses begin to move freely again. Only then should they be removed.

The wearing schedule for soft contact lenses is not as strict as the rigid lens schedule. Generally, day 1 is 4 hours, and each day, an additional 2 hours of wearing time is added.

- Day 1: 4 hours
- Day 2: 6 hours
- Day 3: 8 hours
- Day 4: 10 hours
- Day 5: 12 hours
- Day 6: 14 hours
- Day 7: all waking hours

At the one week follow-up visit, ideally the patient can wear the lenses all day. If the lenses become uncomfortable at the end of the day, they can be removed and rinsed, then reinserted. This rehydrates the lenses and restores the comfort. If the lenses are still uncomfortable, it is probably best to give the eyes a rest and remove the lenses for the rest of the evening. Not all patients can tolerate lenses for the entire day.

Points to remember for soft contact lens wearers include the following:

- Do not switch solutions. Not all solutions are compatible with all contact lens materials. The solutions that are dispensed should be the only ones that are used.

- A damaged lens should not be worn.

- If material gets trapped under a lens, remove and rinse the lens then reinsert it.

- If they have any questions, they should not hesitate to call their practitioner.

Tips for Cosmetics and Contacts Lenses:

- The contacts should be inserted before cosmetics are applied.

- Old cosmetics should not be used since bacterial contamination may be present.

- Do not use other people's cosmetics. Use your own cosmetics and applicators.

- Be careful with hair sprays and spray perfumes; they can adhere to the lens material.

- Do not wear contact lenses in the beauty salon. Hot air from air dryers can irritate the eyes and dry the contacts.

- Avoid oily or powdery types of cosmetics.

- Be careful with nail polish and polish removers. They give off fumes which can damage contact lenses.

- If lenses burn when inserted, they may be contaminated and should be removed and rinsed then reinserted.

Contact Lens Complications

Complications usually result from dirty or damaged lenses or possibly a poorly fitted lens. One of the more common problems with soft contacts, particularly extended wear, is protein and lipid build-up which forms on the surface of the lenses. When this happens, the comfort, vision and wearing time may all be reduced. The only solution is to replace the lenses. The average life span of a soft daily wear lens is about one year and extended wear lenses usually only last about 9 months. Proper cleaning of the lenses with a daily cleaner and a weekly enzyme is necessary to help slow down deposit formations.

An allergic response to these lipid and protein deposits can develop causing inflamed conjunctiva and lens intolerance. Giant papillary conjunctivitis (GPC) is a common allergic response where the conjunctiva react to the eye's own protein build-up. If the condition is very severe, contact lens wear must be discontinued and steroids and other anti-inflammatory agents must be administered. In some cases, contact lens wear must be discontinued permanently.

Another soft contact lens complication is a process called neovascularization. This condition involves tiny abnormal blood vessels growing in a normally vessel free cornea. They are a response to lack of oxygen reaching the cornea. All soft contact lens wearers have some degree of neovascularization, but it usually is insignificant. In severe cases, the patient can be switched to gas permeable (rigid lenses) which allow much more oxygen to reach the cornea.

The most serious complication from soft contact lens wear is a corneal ulcer. A corneal ulcer can be either sterile or from an infection. The eye is usually inflamed, painful and quite sensitive to light. A fast moving ulcer can destroy the cornea and wipe out the vision. It is very important to treat ulcers quickly in order to save the vision. Any eye inflammation or opacity on the cornea should not be taken lightly. At the first sign of discomfort, the contacts should be removed and an eyecare practitioner should be contacted immediately.

A corneal ulcer from an acanthamoeba infection can be particularly devastating. Patients who make up their own saline solution from salt tablets are more susceptible to acanthamoeba infections. These home saline solutions have no preservatives. It is preferable to use store-bought saline, which is either preserved or packaged in a sterile can. Acanthamoeba infections are, fortunately, quite rare.

Contraindications for Contact Lenses

Any of the following conditions can be a contraindication to contact lens use:

- any acute inflammation to the anterior part of the eye
- diabetes
- severe allergic reactions
- dry eye condition
- dirty working environment
- corneal hyposensitivity

The most common drawback to successful contact lens wear is a dry eye problem from insufficient tear production. The lenses dehydrate quickly resulting in discomfort, blurred vision and decreased wearing time. The most susceptible individuals are middle-aged females. Artificial tears can be of some help but may have to be applied frequently.

Types of Contact Lenses

Daily Wear vs. Extended Wear

Daily wear lenses are either soft or rigid lenses which are removed at the end of the day. The patient does not sleep with the lenses. Extended wear lenses can remain in the eye overnight and can be worn for as long as a month, in some cases. In order to make the soft lens acceptable for extended wear, the lens is either made thinner or the water content of the lens is increased. Either of these will increase the oxygen flow through the lens. As a general rule, extended wear lenses are removed weekly and cleaned.

The wearing schedule for extended wear lenses should not exceed the doctor's recommendation.

Most of the eye health complications from contact lenses develop with extended wear patients. The eye is at its most compromised when lenses are worn overnight. With the eyes closed, the cornea swells overnight. During the day (with the eyes open) the cornea returns to its non-swollen state since the oxygen supply to the cornea is greatest when the eyes are open.

More follow-up visits are scheduled for extended wear patients. The eyes must be watched closely for signs of contact lens intolerance. An extended wear schedule is not for everyone. Some people can only tolerate an overnight wearing schedule for a few days, some people one night only and still others cannot sleep with their lenses for even a few hours.

Many patients who attempt an extended wear schedule are forced back into daily wear because of corneal sensitivity or a dry eye condition. People with high prescriptions would likely do best with a daily wear schedule. With high prescriptions, the contacts are thicker and this reduces the amount of oxygen reaching the cornea.

The advantages of an extended wear schedule include instant vision during the night and upon awakening. Also, people with handling difficulties due to physical handicaps such as arthritis, often do well with extended wear.

Extended wear patients are instructed to check for three things when waking up after sleeping with their lenses. They should cover one eye at a time and check their distance vision to make sure things are clear. They should check the appearance of their eyes to make sure they are not red. And they should make sure that the comfort of the lenses is satisfactory. Often eye drops are needed when awakening in order to rehydrate the lenses.

If the extended wear lens patient has discomfort, blurred vision or irritated eyes upon awakening, the contact lenses should be removed until the problem is identified and corrected.

Extended wear lenses are also available in gas permeable (rigid) materials. Gas permeable overnight wear compromises the cornea far less than soft extended wear lenses. There is far less corneal edema and no corneal vascularization. As with soft overnight wear, the major drawback to gas permeable overnight wear is a tendency for the lenses to adhere to the cornea. Rehydrating the lenses upon awakening restores normal lens movement. Overnight wearing of rigid (gas permeable) lenses is a relatively new concept. However, it appears the gas permeable extended contacts are a viable option for selected individuals.

Disposable Contact Lenses

Another new concept in contact lenses is the disposable soft lens. For patients who can tolerate overnight wear, the contacts are worn for a week then removed from the eyes and thrown away. No cleaning or disinfecting solutions are needed, just rehydrating drops.

Many contact lens complications are a result of dirty lenses. Lipid and protein deposits from the tears often soil the lenses leading to discomfort, poor vision and allergic reactions. With disposable lenses, these problems are eliminated. A clean lens is placed on the eye every week.

After the fitting and trial period is over, the patient is given a six month supply of contact lenses. After six months, the patient returns to the practitioner for a follow-up visit and receives the next six month supply of lenses.

After two weeks or so, the integrity of the disposable lens decreases rapidly. This discourages people from overwearing the lenses. Since the lenses are quite expensive, one initial concern was that patients will extend their wearing schedule to save lenses and money. A better alternative to extended wear disposable contacts is daily wear disposables. The lenses are worn as a daily wear lens for two weeks and then discarded. They are simply stored in an overnight disinfecting solution when not being worn. Daily wear

YOUR EYES!

---

disposables are healthier since the lenses are not being worn overnight (extended wear). It is also more economical for patients since they only go through half as many lenses.

Disposable contacts are gaining in popularity with both patients and practitioners and the future of disposable lenses appears bright.

Rigid Lenses for Astigmatism

When high amounts of astigmatic correction are required, either a PMMA or gas permeable lens is necessary. Contact lenses that correct astigmatism are called toric lenses.

Today, few people cannot wear contacts because of astigmatism. Very high amounts can be corrected with a rigid lens called a bitoric lens. It has excellent stability and gives great vision. Bitoric lenses are probably the most sophisticated lenses available; they are custom made and somewhat expensive. But for people who have been told in the past they cannot wear contacts because of their high astigmatism, these lenses are available and work remarkably well.

Patients with moderate amounts of astigmatism who recently tried soft toric lenses and were not happy with their vision, often turn to rigid lenses. Spherical rigid lenses will compensate for small amounts of astigmatism and give crisp vision. Higher amounts need the special toric lenses.

Soft Lenses for Astigmatism

Recent advances in contact lens technology now combine the comfort of soft lenses with corrections for astigmatism. People with high amounts of astigmatism who cannot tolerate rigid lenses for whatever reason now have another option. Soft toric lenses are quite reliable and reproducible and the laboratories guarantee their fit. The lenses are usually weighted to help maintain the proper orientation on the cornea.

The correct orientation is necessary to cancel out the astigmatic error. With the blink, contact lenses rotate but the weighted lens then rotates back to the proper position. This rotation can result in some minimal fluctuating vision. For people who are unhappy with their glasses or never knew that they could wear contacts, this occasional blurred vision is only a minor inconvenience. Soft lenses can also be truncated – the lower part of the lens cut off to help stabilize the lens on the eye.

So basically there are two ways to stabilize astigmatic contacts; either weight the lens at the 6 o'clock position or slice off part of the bottom of the lens (truncation). Both methods will help stabilize the lens resulting in less rotation and more consistent vision. *(Figure 4-11)*

The care and handling instructions for toric lenses are the same as spherical lenses. Because of the expense and the extra time involved in fitting toric lenses, it obviously makes sense to take good care of them.

Bifocal Contact Lenses

There are several bifocal designs available for rigid and soft contact lenses. *(Figures 4-12 and 4-13)* Rigid bifocal contact lenses generally give better vision than soft bifocal contacts. One type of rigid bifocal contact lens has a crescent shaped reading area which comes into focus as the patient looks down. When the patient lowers his eyes, the lense translates (moves) upward allowing the crescent shaped reading area to be used.

A new design is the tangent streak gas permeable bifocal contact lens. The tangent bifocal has the advantage of a gas permeable material as well as the good optics of a rigid lens.

Soft bifocal contacts have three basic designs: 1) the center of the lens is used for near and the periphery of the lens is used for distance, 2) the center of the lens is used for distance and the periphery of the lens is used for near

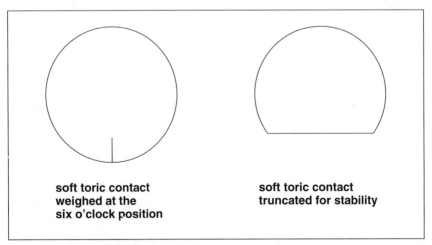

soft toric contact weighed at the six o'clock position

soft toric contact truncated for stability

Figure 4-11   Soft astigmatic contacts.

and 3) the center is used for distance with a gradual increase for near viewing towards the periphery.

A soft bifocal contact lens does not shift with the blink like a rigid lens. Soft bifocal lenses work by a principle called simultaneous vision. When looking up close, the eye looks through the near correction of the lens and the brain will ideally ignore the blur from the distance part of the lens. Conversely, when looking at a distant object, the eye looks through the distance correction of the lens and the brain ignores the blur from the near part of the lens.

Some people cannot tolerate simultaneous vision because their brain cannot tune out the distance blur when looking near and vice versa. For this reason, soft bifocal contacts have limited success. For people who can accept simultaneous vision, soft bifocal lenses free them from glasses throughout their lives and offer the comfort of soft lenses.

A highly successful bifocal contact lens has yet to be invented. The rigid lenses sacrifice comfort for vision and the soft lenses sacrifice vision for comfort. However, some of the newer designs show promise. A breakthrough in contact lens technology will be a boom for the contact lens industry. The aging of the population (particularly the baby-boomers) will greatly increase the market for bifocal contacts in the future.

Tinted Contacts

There are two types of tints for contact lenses: visibility tints and tints that change eye color. Visibility tints are almost always applied to rigid contact

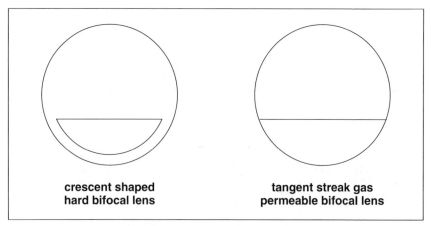

crescent shaped
hard bifocal lens

tangent streak gas
permeable bifocal lens

Figure 4-12 Rigid bifocal designs.

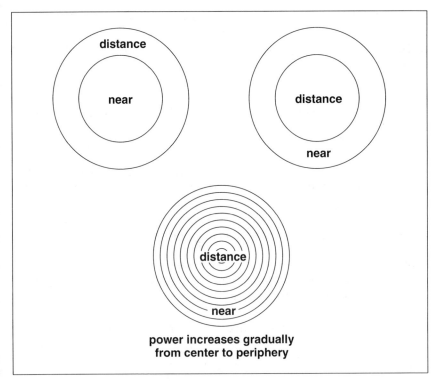

power increases gradually
from center to periphery

Figure 4-13   Soft bifocal designs.

lenses since they are difficult to see when off the eye. They are also available for soft contact lenses. Visibility tints do not change eye color, they just
make handling and cleaning easier and a lost lens with a visibility tint is easier to find.

The second type of contact lens changes eye color. There are two categories of soft color changing contacts: enhancing lenses and opaque color
changing lenses. Enhancing colored contacts are for people with light colored eyes, ideally grey or pale blue. People with grey eyes are the luckiest
because they can change their eye color with enhancing lenses to any color
that they want and look good.

For people with dark eyes who wish to change their eye color they must use
opaque color changing lenses. Nowadays, it is possible to change brown or
very dark eyes to blue, green, aqua, hazel, violet or grey.

The enhancing lenses tend to look more natural than the opaque color changing lenses. The opaque lenses actually have a dot matrix pattern as part of the lens material. When looking very close at the lenses, the normal eye color can be seen "bleeding" through the dot matrix. However, from a distance they look natural.

Tinted lenses are available in extended wear material and astigmatic corrections. Tinted lenses cannot harm the eye in any way and, aside from some possible blurred vision in dim light, have no disadvantages whatsoever.

The patient must have a trial fitting when considering tinted lenses to enhance or change their eye color. Tinted lenses look slightly different on everybody. The lenses may look great on a poster or commercial, but the patient may not like that tint on herself. The only way to tell how tinted lenses will change the overall appearance is to try the lenses.

People with no visual need for contact lenses can also wear tinted lenses if they simply wish to change their eye color. However, they must still take care of the lenses as if they were prescription lenses. Cosmetic tinted lenses, either hard or soft, are available for people who have had eye injuries resulting in pupil or iris abnormalities. These custom made tinted contacts are matched to the patient's normal eye color. They generally give a more natural appearance to the eyes by masking the disfigurement.

Special Cases

Aphakia

Aphakia means the patient has had the lens in the eye removed because of a cataract. Nowadays, implants take the place of the normal lens. In some cases, however, implants cannot be placed in the eye and an aphakic contact lens has to be used. An aphakic contact lens is a high plus lens, +12 for example, that substitutes for the focusing power of the patient's own lens.

Aphakic contact lenses are usually extended wear and can be kept in the eye for several weeks at a time. For some reason, patients who have had the lens of the eye removed seem to have more oxygen reach the cornea. These patients can tolerate an extended wear schedule very nicely.

After cataract surgery, the ideal situation is to have an implant taking the place of the patient's own lens. The next best alternative is an aphakic contact lens. If an implant or contact lens cannot be used, the patient must wear very thick glasses which are neither flattering or optically desirable.

Keratoconus

Keratoconus is a condition in which the cornea becomes excessively steep or curved. The steepening of the apex of the cornea results in thinning and scarring of the corneal tissue. The disease usually begins during the teen years and progresses throughout life. As the severity of the curvature increases, spectacle corrections prove inadequate. Soft contacts are no help since they conform to the irregular shape of the eye. The only solution is a rigid contact lens, usually fit by trial and error.

The rigid lens sometimes slows down the progression of the disease while giving the best possible vision. If the disease progresses to the point where contacts no longer give satisfactory vision, surgery may be required.

Contact Lenses for Infants

Many infants and young children, unfortunately, require contact lenses due to aphakia, a high refractive error or amblyopia. Although contact lenses on infants can be trying for both the practitioner and the parents, eyeglasses are even more impractical.

It is important for infants with severe vision problems to have it corrected or compensated for as soon as possible. The early years are crucial for growth and development and vision plays the major role in this process. Very often contact lenses are the only option.

The major problem with pediatric contact lens wear is keeping the lens on the eye. The infant will very often rub the eye, dislodging or removing the lens. Gas permeable lenses are probably the best choice since they are more difficult to rub out of the eye. The parents must be taught insertion and removal techniques and proper lens care. Only contact lens specialists who work with infants and are comfortable with pediatric patients should be consulted.

Monovision

Monovision is a technique used for presbyopia where one contact lens is fitted for distance viewing and the other is fitted for near viewing. Presbyopia is the gradual loss of near vision that occurs with aging. The monovision

147400

technique is another alternative to bifocal contact lenses and is usually the practitioner's first choice for the presbyopic contact lens wearer. It works surprisingly well and is successful about 70% of the time. When looking up close, the brain tunes out the distance contact and when looking at a distant object, the brain tunes out the near contact. It is a type of simultaneous vision.

The dominant eye is usually fit for distance and the non-dominant eye is fit for near. The eye that you use to look through a camera, for example, is your dominant eye. For most people, it is the right eye.

Monovision, however, has some drawbacks. Some people cannot involuntarily tune out the lens not being used and this results in a visual disturbance. If you cannot adapt to monovision in three weeks, you probably never will and another option must be explored.

Monovision is not ideal for people who have primarily either near demands or distance demands. For example, an accountant would probably not do well with monovision since he does near work all day. A cab driver probably would not do well either since he has primary distance demands. The accountant would be more comfortable visually with reading glasses worn over a pair of contacts for distance. This would allow both eyes to be used for near work. The cab driver would, likewise, do better with both contacts fit for distance and reading glasses to be worn over the contacts for his occasional near demands.

For most people with mixed distance and near demands, monovision works well and is one of the better options available for presbyopic contact lens wearers.

X-Chrome Contact Lens

People with a red-green color deficiency can sometimes have their condition reduced by wearing a red PMMA contact lens over the non-dominant eye. This specialty lens is called the X-Chrome lens.

Individuals with a color deficiency have difficulty distinguishing between different hues of the spectrum. The X-Chrome lens reduces the confusion between colors and helps the wearer distinguish between different shades. The effectiveness of the lens depends on the severity of the condition and the person's response to the lens. It does not work equally well for all individuals and, even with successful cases, much time is required before results can be seen.

Eyeglasses vs. Contact Lenses

Contact lenses offer some distinct advantages over eyeglasses. Cosmetically, people usually look better in contacts as opposed to eyeglasses especially if they have thick lenses. Eyeglasses also cause discomfort on the bridge of the nose and behind the ears. Eyeglasses frequently need adjusting to hold their shape. Furthermore, contact lenses offer better peripheral vision. With eyeglasses, when you glance sideways, the frame and edge of the lens is visible. With contacts, the peripheral vision is clear. Contact lenses, particularly soft contacts, are also ideal for sports and active people. They offer greater comfort and freedom of movement.

Contact lenses sometimes offer a better solution to vision needs than glasses; some refractive errors are better corrected with contacts. Finally, certain eye conditions require a soft bandage contact lens to protect and allow proper healing of the cornea.

YOUR EYES!

5

Visual Disorders Affecting Children & Young Adults

The functional aspects of vision are quite complex. However, the entire visual process can be broken down into two main categories. The first involves getting the visual information to the retina and the second involves processing and interpreting this information. This chapter primarily involves getting the information to the retina for processing. This is called functional vision. The visual stimulus enters the eye and is processed in the retina and is then interpreted by the brain. The physiology and biochemistry of the eye and brain may be intact, but if the visual stimuli never properly reach the retina, the visual process is compromised from the outset.

Many things can affect the visual stimulus and disrupt the flow of visual information. When an object is viewed, the eyes must do two things. They must first align properly with both eyes pointing to the same point, and they must focus on the object being viewed. Any disorder which disrupts proper alignment and/or focusing ability will compromise vision.

Functional vision anomalies are often difficult to diagnose and even more difficult to manage. It is important, however, that they be detected early and corrected. Many learning problems or school difficulties can be attributed to functional anomalies. Many so-called problem children simply have an undetected visual condition.

Convergence Insufficiency

Convergence Insufficiency is a very common misalignment condition; the eyes cannot comfortably converge when viewing a near object. The eyes are diverged outward when viewing a near target. *(Figure 5-1)* About 3% of the population has a Convergence Insufficiency. Symptoms of a Convergence Insufficiency include the following:

- words appear to run together when reading
- after near work, headaches develop
- intermittent double vision with near work
- near blur and sometimes distance blur
- pulling sensation
- heavy eyelids
- loss of concentration

Less common symptoms include the following: nausea, motion sickness, dizziness, general fatigue and poor depth perception. Patients with a Convergence Insufficiency who have these symptoms generally suffer a high amount of anxiety. Prolonged near point activity for these patients can produce nervousness and tension. When the visual discomfort associated with near work is alleviated, the tension is reduced. The anxiety is probably the result of the Convergence Insufficiency, not the cause.

There are many possible causes of a Convergence Insufficiency. One possible cause is a congenital weakness of the medial recti — muscles that allow the eyes to converge. A weakness of these muscles will keep the eyes in an abnormally divergent position causing difficulty with near tasks. Other causes include head trauma and possibly systemic disorders such as mononucleosis or Anemia. In some cases, substance abuse may also be a cause of Convergence Insufficiency. With most cases, however, a cause cannot be found.

The proper management of Convergence Insufficiency is vision therapy. Lenses, prisms and particularly surgery, are not indicated. Vision therapy for Convergence Insufficiency consists of just 5 to 10 visits with the vision therapist.

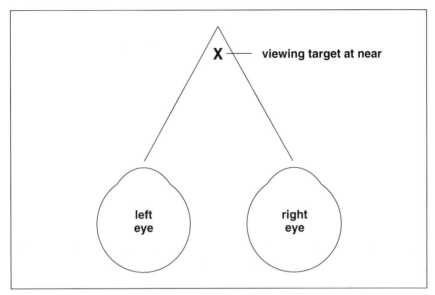

Figure 5-1 Convergence Insufficiency: convergence of the eyes is insufficient and the eyes converge behind the viewing target.

The prognosis with vision training techniques is excellent. With proper vision training, about 90% of Convergence Insufficiency patients are relieved of symptoms and are, in effect, cured of the disorder.

Convergence Excess

Another misalignment condition is Convergence Excess; the eyes are overconverged when viewing a near object. *(Figures 5-2 and 5-3)* This overconvergence places a strain on the visual system. Symptoms of Convergence Excess include the following:

- intermittent blurred vision when viewing near objects
- intermittent double vision when viewing near objects
- eyestrain after prolonged near work
- symptoms are worse at the end of the day

The management of a Convergence Excess is straight-forward: plus lenses, particularly for near viewing. The plus lenses relax the eyes and allow them

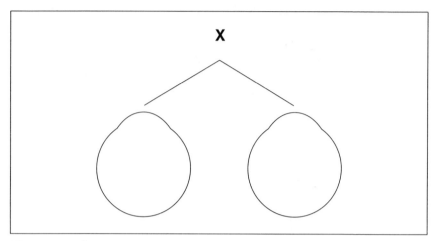

Figure 5-2 Convergence Excess: overconvergence of the eyes with the eyes converging in front of the target.

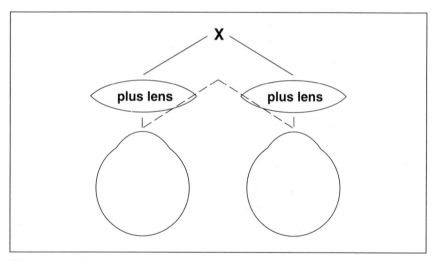

Figure 5-3 Convergence Excess treated with plus lenses. The plus lens prescription allows the eyes to diverge, permitting alignment with the viewing target.

to diverge to a more natural, comfortable position. After receiving the plus lenses, the patient is evaluated again in two months. Although the plus prescription is usually sufficient to eliminate symptoms, visual therapy can be attempted if symptoms persist.

Divergence Insufficiency

Divergence Insufficiency is a misalignment of the eyes when viewing distant objects. The eyes are overconverged and align in front of the viewing target. The symptoms of a Divergence Insufficiency include the following:

- intermittent blur when viewing a distant object
- intermittent double vision when viewing a distant object
- headaches around the eyes
- poor depth perception of distant objects

Treatment of a Divergence Insufficiency includes plus lenses for distance to help relax overconvergence. If this does not work, visual training can be attempted. Divergence Insufficiency is difficult to treat and visual training gives mixed results.

Divergence Excess

Divergence Excess is another misalignment of the eyes when viewing a distant object. The eyes are undercoverged at distance; they cannot converge to the viewing target. The signs of a Divergence Excess include the following:

- person closes one eye in bright light
- parents notice an eye turning out on occasion
- only one eye is used (the other is suppressed) when viewing distant objects

The management of a Divergence Excess can be either surgical or visual training techniques. The first step is to correct any significant refractive error and then attempt visual training. Surgery can always be attempted at a later date. It is difficult to compare the effectiveness of visual training with the effectiveness of surgery. Surgery is strictly a cosmetic cure while visual therapy strives for a functional cure. The various success rates depend on which literature is read. Generally speaking, a functional cure should be attempted first since surgery will not restore binocular function and the surgical success rate is only about 50%.

Convergence Insufficiently, Convergence Excess, Divergence Insufficiency and Divergence Excess are all binocular anomalies where proper alignment of the eyes when viewing a target cannot be achieved comfortably.

Another set of conditions can exist where the alignment of the eyes is fine but the focusing ability is not. These are referred to as accommodative disorders and there are three types: Accommodative Excess, Accommodative Insufficiency and Ill-sustained Accommodation.

When the eye targets an object, the lens changes shape, altering the refractive power of the eye and allowing the object to come into focus. When viewing near objects, the lens has a round shape and when viewing distant objects, the lens has a more oval shape. The lens is constantly changing shape as we look from one object to another. The eye must also focus relatively quick in order to maintain comfortable vision. This focusing usually takes a second or so. This process of rapidly changing focus to meet visual demands is called accommodation.

Accommodative Excess

A patient with an Accommodative Excess has an overactive focusing mechanism which locks in when viewing near objects. When the person tries to view distant objects, the lens of the eye cannot relax and stays focused for near, resulting in distance blur. The Accommodative Excess patient usually holds reading material very close and is often myopic. Symptoms of Accommodative Excess include the following:

- blurred distance vision
- headaches above the eyes after prolonged near work
- general strain around the eyes

Management of an Accommodative Excess involves visual training exercises. The goal is to unlock the near focus and allow the lens to refocus easily when viewing distant objects. Plus lenses for near viewing help the eyes relax. Unfortunately, Accommodative Excess patients cannot accept plus lenses. Visual training techniques help facilitate the focusing ability of the eyes and after successful therapy, the patient can now accept plus lenses for near tasks. This relaxes the eyes and eliminates the symptoms of distance blur and headaches.

Accommodative Insufficiency

When the lens of the eye has difficulty becoming round to allow proper focusing for near objects, this is an Accommodative Insufficiency. It is similar to presbyopia: the inability to focus up close, which begins in the 40s' and gets progressively worse as the person ages. When the inability to focus on near objects is lost at a younger age, it is called Accommodative Insufficiency.

Presbyopia is a normal part of the aging process; Accommodative Insufficiency is an anomaly of the focusing system. Symptoms of an Accommodative Insufficiency include the following:

- blurred near vision
- discomfort and eyestrain after near work
- fatigue after near work

The treatment for an Accommodative Insufficiency is very straight-forward. Plus lenses for near work will alleviate the symptoms and solve the problem nicely.

Accommodative Infacility
(Ill-sustained Accommodation)

The third type of accommodative disorder is Accommodative Infacility which is similar to Accommodative Insufficiency.

The symptoms include the following:

- difficulty focusing from distance to near and near to distance
- near blur
- fatigue with near tasks

Focusing can be achieved, but it takes longer than normal. With a healthy accommodative system, looking at a distant object after prolonged near viewing will take a second or two in order to focus. With an Accomadative Infacility, it may take 10 seconds to focus. The accommodative system works, but it is sluggish.

The treatment consists of visual training exercises which involve rapid visual adjustments from distance to near and near to distance to help facilitate the speed of focusing. The prognosis with visual training is excellent.

As a rule, all of the accommodative disorders respond very nicely to visual training. Daum, in 1983, working at the Ohio State University College of Optometry, assessed 96 patients with accommodative dysfunctions who underwent a visual therapy program. In 53% of the cases, the symptoms were totally eliminated and in 43% of the cases, the symptoms were significantly reduced. The overall success rate for vision therapy was, therefore, 96%.

Amblyopia

Amblyopia (functional) is reduced vision which cannot be corrected by glasses or contact lenses and there is no pathological basis for the vision loss. The central vision is affected in amblyopia, leaving the peripheral vision intact.

If a patient can see the 20/20 line with the right eye and only the 20/40 line with the left eye and the left eye cannot be corrected with refractive lenses, it is amblyopic.

Amblyopia is defined as a significant decrease in acuity in one eye or a significant difference between the acuities of the two eyes. For example, if one eye is 20/15 and the other eye is 20/25, the eye with 20/25 vision is considered amblyopic because there is a significant difference between the acuities of the two eyes.

The amblyopic eye is at its worst with bright illumination. The fovea functions primarily under bright conditions and is also responsible for central vision. The physiological response of the fovea is reduced in amblyopia, decreasing both central vision and reducing acuity in bright light.

Types of Amblyopia

There are two major classifications of amblyopia, functional and organic. Functional amblyopia has no pathological or disease process to explain the reduced vision as opposed to organic amblyopia which has a pathological basis.

Functional Amblyopia

Strabismic Amblyopia

Very often, patients with an eyeturn (strabismus) have amblyopia in the affected eye. The visual image from the deviated eye is suppressed to avoid simultaneous perception of two different objects (double vision). If suppression is long-standing, vision in that eye decreases from lack of use. The peripheral vision remains intact, but central vision becomes reduced.

Refractive Amblyopia (Anisometropic Amblyopia)

This results when the refractive error between the two eyes is unequal. The vision in the eye with the greater refractive error becomes reduced. The vision is reduced in order to avoid interference with the image from the sharper eye.

Stimulus Deprivation Amblyopia (Amblyopia ex Anopsia)

This results when visual acuity is remarkably reduced early in life due to deprivation of visual stimuli. The loss of vision is irreversible. A congenital cataract or anything that prevents visual stimuli from reaching the retina during the critical period of visual development can cause stimulus deprivation amblyopia.

Hysterical Amblyopia

Hysterical amblyopia is an interesting condition where the vision loss is a result of psychological factors. The patient is usually a female around the age of 12. She will complain of blurred distance vision and have no history of vision problems or corrective lenses. The vision loss is bilateral and approximately equal in both eyes. They often have a history of school or emotional problems and a psychological evaluation is in order after a reassurance by the eye doctor that there is no ocular condition present.

Organic Amblyopia

Nutritional Amblyopia

With nutritional amblyopia, the loss of central vision is a result of a deficiency of the B vitamins because of poor dietary habits. It often occurs with alcoholics.

Toxic Amblyopia

The classic case of toxic amblyopia involves ingesting of methyl alcohol. If the amount ingested is not fatal, it will leave the patient with a bilateral, deep loss of central vision.

Congenital Amblyopia

The reduced central vision is a result of a congenital or hereditary anomaly in the visual receptors or visual pathway. Very often, these children have other vision problems such as reduced color vision, nystagmus(jerky eye movements) or high refractive errors. Congenital amblyopia is usually bilateral.

Strabismus

A strabismus, also called a squint or a tropia, is a misalignment of one of the eyes. It is the most serious of functional disorders since no binocular vision can be present with a strabismus. The eye turn can be inward or outward (horizontal) or up or down (vertical). *(Figure 5-4)* Very often, a horizontal and vertical component can be present in the same eye; the eye can deviate up and outward, for example.

A person with a strabismus has no stereopsis or depth perception (a strabismic could not appreciate the visual effects of a 3D movie). Difficulty with depth perception becomes more pronounced at night and driving a car can become particularly difficult for strabismic patients. Judging the distance between your car and other moving vehicles requires good depth perception.

Strabismus that is present before 6 months of age is congenital; after 6 months it is considered acquired.

The eyeturn can be present all of the time (constant) or intermittent. If the eyeturn is present 95% of the time, it is considered intermittent. Intermittent eye deviations have a better prognosis.

The strabismus can also be either unilateral or alternating. Unilateral deviations are always the same eye while alternating deviations switch from one eye to the other. With alternating deviations, the right eye can be turned in towards the nose and the left eye remains straight. The situation can then reverse with the left eye turned in towards the nose and the right eye now straight.

An eye turning in towards the nose is called an esotropia. An eye turning outward is called an exotropia. An eye pointed upward is called a hypertropia. An eye pointed down is not called a hypotropia. The vertical component is labeled by the higher eye. For example, if the right eye is lower than the left eye, the condition is called a left hypertropia (not a right hypotropia).

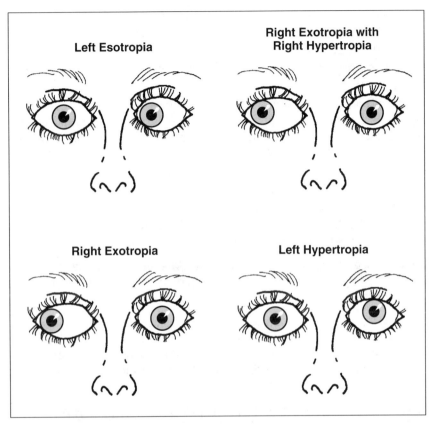

Left Esotropia

Right Exotropia with
Right Hypertropia

Right Exotropia

Left Hypertropia

Figure 5-4 Examples of strabismus.

A right eye turned in towards the nose, present all of the time and always the same eye, would be called a constant, unilateral right esotropia.

An eyeturn outward that is not present all of the time and switches from one eye to the other is called an intermittent, alternating exotropia. Usually, alternating tropias have a dominating eye where, for example, the right eye may deviate 70% of the time and the left eye deviates only 30% of the time. When the one eye is deviated, the other eye remains straight.

Alternating, intermittent eyeturns are usually less detrimental than unilateral, constant ones. When one eye is deviated constantly, the vision in that eye may decrease over time since that eye is not being used. The central vision will decrease (amblyopia). However, an alternating eyeturn will not result in amblyopia because both eyes will be used, although not at the same time. An eye that is deviated 70% of the time will, obviously, be straight 30% of the time. Even when the eye is used only 30% of the time, amblyopia will not develop because there will be enough visual stimulation to keep the vision intact.

Almost all congenital eyeturns are esotropias (eye turns inward); exotropias (eye turns outward) are acquired after six months of age. Esotropia usually results in amblyopia and exotropia usually results in suppression of the visual image of the deviated eye.

Both amblyopia and suppression achieve the same result: they prevent the brain from seeing two images, one from the deviated eye and one from the straight eye. Seeing double is extremely uncomfortable. The brain compensates by either blurring the vision of the deviated eye (amblyopia) or tuning out the vision not being used (suppression).

In either case, there is a loss of binocularity. Patients with a tropia cannot use both of their eyes at the same time. Depth perception and distance judgement, therefore, suffer.

Binocularity (using both eyes simultaneously) is vision that is functionally intact. Vision therapy attempts to restore binocularity (functional vision) by overcoming the suppression or reducing the amblyopia. It is not always successful and requires much time and patience, but the goal of establishing functional vision is well worth the effort.

When the deviation cannot be reduced by vision therapy (the suppression is too embedded or the angle of the deviation is too large), cosmetic surgery can be attempted. Surgery is strictly a cosmetic cure and does nothing to restore binocularity. The amblyopia or suppression will still exist after surgery. Sometimes, vision therapy is done first to restore some binocularity and then surgery is performed to improve the cosmetic appearance.

A good prognosis for a functional cure depends on several factors. Ideally, the patient should be between 7 and 11 years of age and cooperative enough to attempt vision therapy. An intermittent tropia is more favorable than a constant one. Exotropes do better in therapy than esotropes and patients with small angle deviations do better than patients with large deviations. Esotropes who suppress or who have significant amblyopia are also poor candidates for a functional cure.

Evaluating strabismus, suppression and amblyopia is one of the more complex aspects of vision care. The family history is important as well as the child's developmental history. The time of onset, the duration and the magnitude of the eyeturn must all be evaluated. Any accompanying visual problems must also be evaluated, such as nystagmus, which could indicate that a syndrome is present.

The work-up for a strabismic patient is extensive and time consuming. An optometrist specializing in pediatric care should be consulted when a strabismus is suspected. A pediatric optometrist deals only with functional vision problems and together with the pediatric ophthalmologist (surgeon) can determine the best course of action.

When a deviation is noted by the examining doctor, it must be established whether it is of recent onset or it has been present for many years. A recent onset tropia must be followed by a complete medical and neurological evaluation to rule out eye disease or injury.

Frequently, the doctor will request some old photographs of the patient. The old photographs may reveal the presence of an abnormal head posture or the tropia itself eliminating the possibility of a recent onset. A recent onset tropia, often accompanied by double vision, may be a medical emergency and must be examined vigorously.

Recent onset tropias are often caused by damage to one of the extraocular muscles or one of the cranial nerves supplying the eye. The tropia is called paralytic; the result of a partial or complete impairment of the motor function of the eye. Damage to the muscle or the nerve supplying the muscle prevents the eyes from working together as a team. This results in double vision.

Many factors or conditions can cause a paralytic tropia. Some of the more common causes are listed below:

- diabetes
- head trauma
- nerve palsy
- disease of the muscle itself
- orbital fractures
- scar formation around the muscle following repeated eye surgery
- aneurysm
- intracranial neoplasm (tumor)

Treatment Methods for Binocular Anomalies

Occlusion Therapy

Occlusion is primarily used to treat amblyopia. It can also be used for suppression, strabismus and diplopia (double vision). Occlusion therapy is quick, easy to administer and inexpensive. With amblyopia, the "good" eye is covered with a patch to force the amblyopic eye to work. The occlusion is usually only several hours a day and visual exercises are given when the patch is on in order to stimulate the weaker eye. It is not a good idea to patch the good eye for prolonged periods of time since the vision in that eye will then become reduced because of lack of stimulation.

Patching the stronger eye is called direct occlusion. Direct occlusion can also be attempted in strabismic cases to help develop fixational abilities. It is also used to stimulate hand eye coordination by covering the good eye and forcing the strabismic eye to take up the slack.

Sometimes, it is not good to occlude all light from reaching an eye and a non-opaque occluder is used. A non-opaque occluder allows some light to enter the eye but blurs things significantly.

Occluders can be patches which are either opaque or polarized filters, frosted lenses or contact lenses. In addition, the occlusion can be either full, covering the eye completely, or partial, with just a portion of the visual field covered.

Occlusion can be used for preventing suppression by occluding the non-suppressed eye and is also used for double vision by preventing binocularity. Because of the visual discomfort associated with double vision, an eye is often occluded to relieve the symptoms while the cause of the diplopia is being investigated.

Lenses

Lenses have been used for years to compensate for binocular anomalies. It is important to correct any significant refractive error at an early age since poor uncorrected vision can lead to amblyopia. Corrections for astigmatism are important to allow visual acuity to develop normally. If an eye has a large amount of astigmatism, the child may develop amblyopia if the eye remains uncorrected.

Prisms

Prisms are used to deviate light and re-direct the image of the incoming stimuli. They are occasionally used for children with strabismus and are incorporated into their eyeglasses. Prisms can sometimes improve the alignment of the eyes and can also enhance the cosmetic appearance of the child. The benefits are limited, however, and the results are often transient requiring other treatment methods.

Extraocular Muscle Surgery

Surgery is attempted when the cosmetic appearance of the patient is a consideration or when the angle of the deviation is too great to attempt a functional cure. If vision therapy is not practical, possibly because of the patient's age, surgery is also recommended.

The main approach to cosmetic surgery on the extraocular muscles is either to strengthen or weaken a muscle. A recession procedure weakens the muscle by moving the insertion of the muscle to a different location, lessening its mechanical action.

A resection procedure strengthens the muscle by shortening it. This gives the muscle greater mechanical action.

In esotropic cases (eye turns inward), a recession procedure is done on the medial rectus muscle. The medial recti muscles turn the eyes inward. This procedure weakens the muscle forcing the eye outward. In exotropia cases (eye turns outward), a recession procedure is done on the lateral rectus muscle. The lateral recti muscles turn the eyes outward . This procedure weakens the muscle forcing the eye inward. A resection of the medial rectus muscle can also be done with high exotropia to strengthen the muscle that helps turn the eye inward.

Congenital esotropia (present before six months of age) requires surgical alignment of the eyes. Any non-surgical treatment is directed towards correcting any refractive error that may be present. Children with CONGENITAL esotropia should have surgery as soon as possible. The eyes will not align spontaneously and waiting until the pre-school years before operating may cause irreversible vision loss.

Most surgeons prefer to operate on a congenital esotropia when the child is two years of age or possibly older. They will not operate during infancy, generally. The surgery is primarily for an improved cosmetic appearance although with later therapy some binocular function can be obtained.

After the surgery, there is often a small angle deviation which does not look bad cosmetically. However, the eyes will not be functioning as a team and there may be suppression in one eye and no stereopsis (depth perception). The eyes may look "cured" but functional vision will not be present. The post-operative care involves preventing amblyopia from developing and correcting any refractive error which may be present.

A study of 100 patients who had surgery for congenital esotropia (the Wilmer study and the Washington study) reveals the following: a perfect alignment was achieved in 7 cases and an acceptable deviation (small angle) was achieved in 60 cases. (modified from von Noorden).

With congenital exotropia (eye turns outward noticed prior to 6 months of age), surgery is also recommended. The surgery is performed between the ages 1 and 2. In adults with large angle deviations, surgery is performed to improve the cosmetic appearance. If the deviation has been present since childhood, the prognosis for normal binocular function is poor. Furthermore, the decision to operate depends on the size of the deviation. A small deviation (cosmetically acceptable) will not require an operation.

Some binocular function may be restored after surgery to align the eyes. If the exotropia is long-standing and constant, the prognosis for a functional cure following surgery is poor.

Vision Therapy

Vision therapy is a teaching and training process for the improvement of eye coordination and the achievement of more efficient and comfortable binocular vision. Training can help the patient regain lost visual skills or develop skills that have been arrested. Vision therapy is a functional cure, not strictly cosmetic.

According to Flom, the criteria for functional cure include the following:

- clear, comfortable, single binocular vision
- stereopsis must be present (depth perception)
- normal ranges of motor fusion (eye movements in various directions and can still maintain binocular vision)

The goal of vision therapy (training) is to attempt to restore normal, comfortable vision, alleviating the patient's symptoms.

The non-strabismic binocular disorders (Convergence Insufficiency, for example) can be modified by optometric vision therapy to a significant extent. These disorders may not be a cosmetic problem, but they can seriously impair productivity by disrupting reading and other near-point activities. Visual concentration and the processing of information can be compromised. Learning can, therefore, be affected.

Accommodative disorders also respond very nicely to vision therapy. After therapy, symptoms are reduced and accommodative facility is restored. The speed and accuracy of the eye's focusing ability is improved.

The binocular system and the accommodative system interact in normal functioning vision. For example, when a near object is viewed, the eyes must change focus (accommodate) to view the object clearly and the eyes must converge (binocular adjustment). Very often, a disorder of the binocular system has an accompanying accommodative problem. A Convergence Insufficiency disorder frequently involves an Accommodative Insufficiency as well. The eyes can neither converge to view a near object nor can they focus properly on the object.

Visual training procedures incorporate both binocular and accommodative exercises. One or the other may be stressed during the program, depending on the dysfunction, but both will be incorporated into the training regimen.

The Visual Training Program

Usually, a visual training program consists of both home training and in-office training. The office training can be weekly and the home training is often several times a week. Sometimes, home-based training is not recommended because the patient is too young or because the parents cannot monitor the child's home training program. If the dysfunction is severe, only office procedures are attempted.

The patient is provided with a set of instructions for home training as well as a schedule. The child will be asked to demonstrate the task before leaving the office. They will also be provided with a calender to help chart their progress. When the child returns to the office for training or progress evaluations, a history update is given to determine if symptoms have improved. The patient will be asked to demonstrate the training task; appropriate changes in the program will be made by the doctor.

It is important that the patient can achieve the objective in any particular task. If the training exercise is too difficult and cannot be accomplished, the child will lose interest and motivation.

The key to successful vision therapy is motivation. A child that is not motivated will not persevere throughout the training exercises. If a child has no symptoms, therapy can be difficult. A patient who has visual discomfort will be more willing to undergo visual therapy since his goal will be comfortable vision and the loss of symptoms.

The in-office therapy sessions usually last about 45 minutes and the therapist will monitor the vision therapy to insure that the proper technique is being used. The home therapy is generally for repetition of developed skills. Usually, only one or two techniques are sent home with the child to insure that he is not overwhelmed by the training material.

Vision Therapy Techniques

Listed below are samples of a few vision training techniques used during therapy. There are literally hundreds of techniques and devices which can be used for training purposes. The training program is tailored specifically for each individual and is modified during the course of treatment. The stages of training become progressively more challenging as some techniques are dropped and others added. The goal, hopefully accomplished at the end of the therapy, is clear, comfortable, binocular vision under all conditions.

The Brock String

The Brock String is a long white cord with two or three movable wooden beads. It is used primarily for Convergence Insufficiency. The purpose is to create an awareness of converging the eyes.

One end of the string is attached to a wall and the other end is held taut against the patient's nose. When one of the beads is fixated, the others will appear double. This is normal and called physiological diplopia. Also, it should appear as if two strings are crossing at the point of fixation. The strings will form an "X" at this bead. The patient is asked to look from a more distant bead to a bead closer on the string. With both eyes open, if one of the strings appears to disappear, this means that both eyes are not being used together. Rapid blinking should bring the "X" pattern back at the fixating bead. The "X" pattern should be maintained for a count of 10 seconds.

The patient is then asked to quickly shift from the near bead to the far bead and back again. This works the accommodative system as well as the convergence system.

As these tasks become easy, the near bead is pushed closer up the string towards the patient's nose. The exercises are then repeated. The patient is reminded to try to get the feeling that the eyes are converging and that they are looking closer.

The near bead is moved closer to the nose, two inches at a time, until the exercises can be performed with the bead only one inch from the nose. The patient must be aware of the act of converging the eyes during the exercise.

Teaching convergence (to overcome a Convergence Insufficiency) is one of the more common training techniques. It is quick and easy and is quite successful. The Brock String exercise is just one example of a convergence training technique. It can be incorporated easily into both home and in-office procedures.

The Aperture Rule

A more sophisticated training procedure (for both convergence and divergence problems) is the aperture rule. *(Figure 5-5)*

The double aperture window (two side-by-side slits) is used to teach convergence of the eyes and the single aperture is used to teach divergence of the eyes. With convergence training, the patient must get the feeling of looking close and crossing the eyes. With divergence training, the patient must get the feeling of relaxing the eyes and looking far away. The aperture rule can be quite challenging, particularly the divergence training.

Aperture rule training cards are used with either the single aperture or the double aperture depending on whether divergence or convergence is desired. The cards have identical images, side by side. One image will have a tiny cross on it and the other identical image will have a dot on it. When the images are merged as one, both the dot and the cross must remain visible. This insures binocular vision throughout the exercise. The more difficult the exercises, the further the images are apart on the cards.

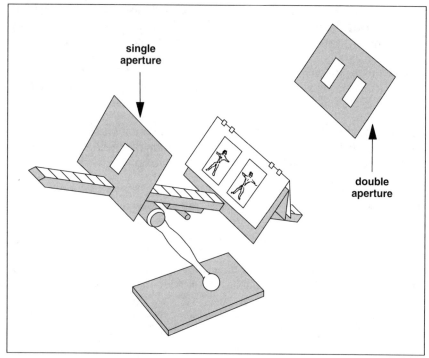

Figure 5-5 Aperture rule.

The following is a description of convergence training (double aperture). Looking with both eyes open, the patient attempts to merge the two targets into one. The target should appear clear and single and both the dot and the cross must remain visible. The image of the target is maintained for 20 seconds and the dot and the cross must be noticed at all times. The patient then looks elsewhere for a few seconds and then looks back to the target trying to maintain the single image for 20 seconds. This activity is repeated 10 times.

Usually, about 10 to 15 minutes are devoted to the aperture rule at any session. As the session progress, the more difficult cards are attempted. The aperture rule is not used in the early training sessions; it is too difficult for the beginning stages of the vision training program.

The Eccentric Rings

This is a free-space technique in which no instrument is required. It is attempted after the patient masters the aperture rule. The eccentric rings can be used for either divergence or convergence training using the same cards. The patient just uses his eyes differently. *(Figure 5-6)*

Divergence Training

Position the two cards at arm's length. The cards should be edge to edge and at the same height. They should be the same distance from the eyes with the "A's" together. A pointer is held midway between the cards and the eyes. With only the right eye open, the pointer should be centered over the left card and with the left eye open, the pointer should be centered over the right card.

With both eyes open, the patient looks at the tip of the pointer. He will see three cards instead of two. The middle card will have a "stereo" effect. The goal is to maintain the middle card clearly noting the stereo effect. The patient looks away and then back to the cards again, trying to recover the same effect. The exercise is repeated 10 times.

When this exercise is mastered, it is attempted without the pointer. When this condition can be maintained, the cards are slowly brought closer to the patient while continuing to focus on the middle card. The cards are then separated by an inch. The patient maintains focus on the middle card. As the cards are separated, they will appear to move closer and become smaller. As the patient becomes more proficient, the cards are gradually moved closer to the patient and the separation between them is increased.

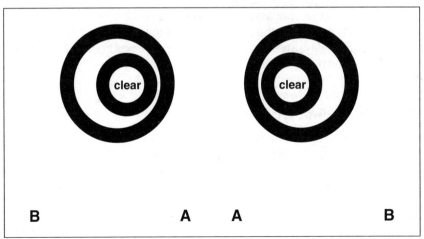

B   **A   A**   **B**

Figure 5-6 Eccentric rings.

The eccentric rings are one of the more difficult vision training devices. They are usually incorporated much later in the training program.

The Hart Card

The Hart Card is used to treat the accommodative system. It consists of two identical charts; one has small print and the other has large print. The big chart is placed 10 feet away on a wall. The small chart is held at arm's length and, keeping the top line clear, the chart is slowly moved closer. When the top line blurs, the patient switches fixation from the near chart to the far chart on the wall. He reads the second line on the far chart. He then switches back and reads the third line on the near chart. The patient alternates back and forth from far to near until the chart is finished. The exercise is repeated several times.

The exercise is performed one eye at a time. A patch is placed over the eye not being used. Any exercise working the accommodative system must be done monocularly. If both eyes are used together, the convergence system will come into play.

There are many variations of the Hart Chart technique for accommodative training. Sometimes, plus or minus lenses are placed over the eye that is being trained to make the exercise more difficult. The Hart Chart is just one example of an accommodative technique. It is easy to perform and can be done both at home and in the office. The accommodative system responds very nicely to training and the success rate of accommodative dysfunctions with vision therapy is quite high.

Therapy for Amblyopia

Amblyopia is reduced vision, usually in only one eye, which cannot be corrected with glasses or contact lenses. Amblyopia that responds to vision therapy will not have an organic basis (caused by a disease or structural defect). If the amblyopia is organic in nature, therapy will be of no help. The basic treatment for non-organic amblyopia is occlusion therapy. The good eye is patched and this forces the amblyopic eye to work. The occlusion is usually just for a few hours at a time. Various visually demanding tasks are performed during the occlusion period in order to stimulate the weaker eye.

The following is a list of activities for the infant (under 2) with amblyopia during occlusion therapy. The stronger eye is patched.

- peek-a-boo games
- catching a rolling ball
- handling toys
- watching toys suspended from above
- playing with bright objects
- watching television

The following list of activities is for patients over the age of 2:

- balancing exercise (walking on balance beam)
- running, hopping
- throwing and catching a ball
- drawing and coloring
- dot-to-dot pictures
- tracing
- crossword puzzles

(modified from Griffin)

There are hundreds of visually stimulating exercises which can be performed to help improve the acuity of an amblyopic eye. The exercises, with an eye patched, can be done at home and at therapy sessions.

The patching is done on a part-time basis because prolonged patching of the good eye can reduce vision in that eye. After months of therapy, if the treatment is successful, the visual acuity in the amblyopic eye will improve. Amblyopic therapy is recommended because it cannot hurt the situation and may help.

The younger the patient, the better the chance for improvement. It was previously believed that if amblyopia therapy was not performed before the age of seven, it had no chance of success. New evidence suggests that the therapy can be successful in older children and even adults. When a disease process has been ruled out, amblyopia therapy is certainly a viable option in attempting to restore vision in a weak eye.

Perceptual Deficiencies

Perception is the process of using our senses to analyze the environment and make sense of that information. The information is brought to the brain for processing and interpretation. The five senses (taste, hearing, smell, sight and touch) allow the information to be assessed. Visual function (sight) brings the information to the retina where it is processed and then interpreted in the brain. Sight would be spotting an open manhole; perception would be interpreting the information and having enough sense to walk around it.

Perceptual deficiencies may be noted in a child who cannot "keep up" with his peers. The child's rate of development is too slow. The child may not have any physical or intellectual problems but may have perceptual lags. When tested, he may perform lower than his chronological age would indicate. Normal perceptual skills fit into a range where most of the child's peers will fall.

A child with a perceptual problem will have a history of poor academics or poor performance at sports or hobbies. He just cannot quite keep pace with his peers in schoolwork, sports, etc.

There are many sophisticated tests available to the specialist to analyze perceptual deficiencies. Perception can be broken down into specific categories.

The basic areas of visual perception are as follows:

- bilateral integration and gross motor skills (coordination involving opposite sides of the body)
- organizational abilities and visual motor integration (hand/eye coordination)
- directionality (distinguishing right from left)
- auditory visual integration (integrating what is heard with what is seen)
- visual perception and attention skills (these skills include form perception, figure ground skills, visual closure, visual sequencing and visualization).

A child with poor bilateral integration and gross motor skills will usually lack balance and coordination. He will often do poorly in athletics and tends to play with younger children. In addition, he will have a tendency to bump into objects and cannot sit still. The child will also favor one side of his body when performing rhythmic activities.

A child with poor hand-eye coordination (visual motor integration) will tend to have poor handwriting skills and will have difficulty staying within the lines when drawing. The child responds well orally but does poorly in written tests.

He has a tendency to use his hand to keep his place when reading. Furthermore, the child erases excessively when doing written work and has difficulty following written instructions.

Directionality means distinguishing right from left and the concept usually develops around the age of seven. Reversing letters and/or words when writing is the classic sign of a directionality problem. In addition, the child will have difficulty distinguishing right from left, past the age of seven.

Auditory visual problems are often present with poor spelling ability and difficulty sequencing material presented verbally. The child cannot follow verbal instructions and can have a problem relating symbols to their sounds. Furthermore, the child with auditory visual perceptual difficulties often mistakes words that are similar when presented verbally.

Difficulties with visual perceptual discrimination (attention skills) can present a myriad of signs.

Difficulty with form perception:

- may be a problem recognizing the alphabet
- may mistake words that have similar beginnings
- problem recognizing the same word on the same page

Difficulty with figure ground:

- has a tendency not to complete work
- not aware of what should be attended to
- cannot separate what is significant from what is insignificant when performing tasks

Difficulty with visual closure:

- may perform slowly when doing visual tasks
- can perform parts of the task but cannot put them together
- usually shows poor comprehension

Difficulty with visual sequencing:

- has a problem with organizing materials
- has a problem placing visual information into categories
- difficulty with procedures requiring more than one step

Difficulty with visualization:

- problem learning new material
- problem anticipating next step in a visual task
- cannot visualize what is read
- cannot recall material presented visually
- has a tendency to avoid new learning situations

When analyzing perceptual problems, it is important to realize that not every child can be strong in every category. There are perceptual tests available designed to measure development and these are compared to the normal development of children of the same age.

The child's behavior is also watched carefully and, together with the test results, an assessment of the perceptual areas can be made. When the weak areas are determined, appropriate treatment can be initiated. Various perceptual exercises can be performed during vision therapy. The training is an attempt to strengthen the child's perceptual development.

It is obviously important to identify and help correct perceptual problems since learning can be compromised. Very often, a pediatric vision clinic will include specialists from the fields of optometry, education and psychology. Assessing perceptual and/or learning difficulties is not an easy task. Analyzing human behavior is a tricky business and is hardly an exact science. But the effort should be made since the child's development and overall well-being are at stake.

Normal Developmental Stages in Children

The following stages represent the normal course of child development. Every child will not reach every stage at the same time. If a child is not performing a particular behavior at the time that most children are, it is no reason to be concerned. The actual time that the behavior develops is not as important as the developmental sequence. The behavior is learned in steps.

Some children will be ahead in some areas and behind in others. However, if the child lags in several areas of developmental behavior, that may be significant.

- 4 weeks   infant's head momentarily lifts up
- 6 weeks   binocular vision develops
- 16 weeks   laughter develops
- 24 weeks   baby holds bottle
- 13 months   baby first walks
- 2 years   child runs
- 3 years   normal speech develops; child can copy a circle
- 4 years   child can copy a cross
- 5 years   child can copy a triangle

Fixation

- birth   crude eye movements, eyes move independently
- 1 month   child can fixate object but must alternate eyes
- 2 months   binocular fixation, only occasionally
- 3 months   part time binocular fixation
- 6 months   binocular fixation is pretty well established

Tracking (the baby follows movement)

- at birth   only very large objects can be tracked: eyes only move about 45 degrees
- one month   large objects can be tracked with eye movements up to 90 degrees
- two months   child can follow small objects with eye movements up to 150 degrees
- three months   small objects can be followed up to 180 degrees

Reaching and Grasping (hand/eye coordination)

- one month   very little grasping
- two months   child looks at his hand for a few seconds

- 2¹/₂ months   child begins to swipe at objects
- three months   child's hands can move toward the midline
- 3¹/₂ months   child can grasp objects for a few seconds
- four months   when an object is presented at the midline, the child can grasp it with both hands
- 4¹/₂ months hand   the child can reach up and grasp an object with one
- five months   child can reach up and grasp an object without looking at his hand. Previously, the child had to look at his hand when reaching up to grasp an object.

Directional Development

- 0-3 years of age   the child cannot distinguish between right and left
- 4-7 years of age   right and left are known to be on opposite sides of the body, but cannot be identified
- after 7 years of age   right and left can be differentiated

Sensory Motor Development

- less than 1 month   child is unaware of himself or objects
- 1-4 months   child can look around and grasp things
- 4-8 months   child can manipulate some objects but cannot control things. (The child places an object in his mouth a lot during this stage).
- 8-12 months   child can recall some objects (memory) but has no constancy of space. For example, if a toy is placed under a pillow with the child watching, the child will retrieve the object. Now if the toy is placed under a different pillow, the child will search under the first pillow because he cannot yet transfer space.
- 12-15 months   a concept of time develops. The child is aware that certain television programs are aired at specific times.
- 15-24 months   abstract thoughts begin to form; the child can separate from his parents. Before this stage,

	when the parent was out of sight, they did not exist to the child.
• 2-7 years	language develops. The ability to label things also develops. Memory recall is also present.
• 7-11 years	mathematical skills develop
• 11-15 years	abstract logic develops including problem solving ability

Symptoms of Sensory Motor Problems

Sensory

- child has loss of depth perception (stereopsis)
- one eye does not see as clear as the other
- child may turn head at an angle in order to get clear vision

Motor

- skipping lines when reading
- jumping words when reading
- frequent loss of place when reading
- excessive head movements during reading

Allergic Conditions

In any given population, allergic conditions can be found in 15 to 20% of the group. There is usually a strong family history of allergies; the more family members who have allergies, the more likely that an individual will also have them.

An allergy is a hypersensitivity response to a substance found normally in the environment. It usually takes three months for this sensitivity to develop. The hypersensitivity response is an inflammatory one characterized by redness, swelling and itching.

Parents should expect an allergic condition if the following signs are present in a child:

- puffiness under the lids
- an itchy nose

- a purplish discoloration around the eyes
- the child has his mouth open all the time for breathing because of nasal obstruction
- chronically inflamed tissue adjacent to the nose as a result of sinus congestion

An allergy specialist should be consulted since tracking down the offending substance can be difficult. Many medications can be used to help alleviate the symptoms of an allergic response. The best solution, although not always practical, is to remove the offending substance. Airborne substances (pollen, dust) cannot be eliminated and reducing the symptoms may be all that is possible. Hypersensitivity shots may also be attempted if the allergist thinks that it might be beneficial.

Down's Syndrome

Down's Syndrome is the most common cause of mental retardation. It is a genetic condition where chromosome #21 is a triplet instead of a pair. Normally, there are 23 pairs of chromosomes giving a total of 46. A child with Down's Syndrome will have a total of 47 chromosomes instead of 46.

The incidence of Down's Syndrome is 1 in 660 live births. Women over the age of 35 who are having their first child, have a higher incidence of producing a child with Down's Syndrome compared to other women. Recent studies suggest that if the man is much older than the woman, the incidence is also higher.

Down's Syndrome patients resemble each other more than they do their own family members. They usually have fair complexions and blue eyes. They have heavy, large necks and light straight hair. They also have a rising slant to their eyes and a flat nose bridge. In addition, they frequently have irregular shaped teeth and the tips of their ears are folded over.

There are many eye complications associated with Down's Syndrome. Some or all of the following may be present:

- cataracts
- droopy lids (ptosis)
- white specks over the iris
- nystagmus (jerky eye movements)

- strabismus
- hyperopia
- high amounts of astigmatism

Down's Syndrome children obviously need special attention and the primary care optometrist will direct the parents to the appropriate specialists. With proper care and treatment, the Down's Syndrome child can often lead a reasonably normal and happy life.

YOUR EYES!

6

Sports Vision and Environmental Eyecare

I. Sports Vision

Sports vision is a specialty of optometry. It includes providing eye protection, vision training and the prescribing of special lenses for athletes. It also includes fitting contact lenses for sports wear. Optometrists who specialize in sports vision are often consultants for sports teams.

Sports vision has been a recognized specialty for only about fifteen years. Recently, it has been gaining acceptance among sports professionals and enthusiasts.

The training aspect of sports vision is based on the premise that many athletic problems have a visual basis. Such visual abilities as depth perception, peripheral awareness and dynamic visual acuity are linked to athletic performance. Sports vision experts believe that these visual skills are trainable.

The athlete who is not reaching his potential or who consistently has trouble with specific skills can benefit from a sports vision training program. Problems with concentration or technique can often be traced to a visual breakdown.

YOUR EYES!

Athletes have better visual skills than non-athletes. They generally have a larger visual field and their peripheral awareness is greater. They also have better depth perception and better dynamic visual acuity. Athletes also track objects faster and with greater accuracy than non-athletes. The better the athlete, the better the visual skills. The weaker athletes have poorer visual skills than the superior athletes but better skills than the non-athlete.

The Visual Skills Needed for Sports

Dynamic visual acuity measures how well an individual can see a moving target. Since most sports involve motion, the enhancement of this skill is, obviously, important. Dynamic visual acuity correlates very well with a sport such as basketball, for example. A superior ability to accurately spot moving targets and respond accordingly is a great asset to the basketball player.

Dynamic visual acuity also plays a significant role in any sport where an object is projected at a player, such as tennis or baseball. In baseball, the hitter must track the pitched ball, maintaining a clear focus on the moving target. This type of visual acuity is much different from static visual acuity such as reading an eye chart. A person can have 20/20 vision, as measured by an eye chart, but their dynamic visual acuity can be deficient. This individual will have difficulty hitting a baseball, for example.

The training of dynamic visual acuity is an important part of any sports vision program. This is particularly important for athletes involved in sports where moving objects are projected either towards or away from the individual.

Another important visual skill for the athlete is depth perception. The binocular visual system, when functioning properly, allows three dimensional viewing of objects. Depth perception, which is related to stereopsis, is exceptionally acute in the athlete. Depth perception is extremely important when shooting a basketball. Next time on the court, try shooting a basketball with one eye closed. The shots will either fall short or hit beyond the rim. Without both eyes open together, most clues to distance and depth are wiped out.

Depth perception is also important when judging approaching objects. A shortstop fielding a ground ball must judge the distance between the bounces in order to make the play. The centerfielder must judge the speed and trajectory of a flyball before positioning himself underneath it.

Impairment of depth perception can result from the eyes either overconverging or underconverging. Any misalignment of the eyes can reduce the stereoscopic effect of binocular vision. When the condition is correctly identified, vision training exercises can help alleviate the problem and improve depth perception. The individual's athletic performance will consequently improve.

Eye/hand/body coordination is how the body responds to visual information. Overall performance is affected since body control and timing are involved. If the visual information is not accurate, timing will be off and the performance level will drop. Better coordination between eyes and body can also be improved with practice.

Another area of importance is visual concentration. This refers to the controlling of the visual system for better awareness. Visual concentration blocks out distractions and allows focusing on the situation at hand.

As a general rule, the shorter the period of time a person concentrates visually, the more intense the concentration. If the activity takes too long, such as an easy catch in football, the mind tends to wander and the ball is often dropped. On the other hand, a very difficult catch in football requires great visual concentration over a shorter period of time.

Ocular motility refers to eye movements needed to track an object and keep it in focus. Slow eye movements are called pursuits and are used primarily for the steady tracking of an object.

Rapid eye movements are called saccades and are often used in sports to quickly pick up fast moving objects. With saccadic eye movements, the eyes must constantly converge and diverge at a high speed.

Studies have shown that baseball hitters, when tracking a pitched ball, use pursuit movements while keeping the head steady. The ball is not tracked all the way to the bat, however. The visual system breaks down at very high velocities and tracking of the pitched ball cannot be followed at very close distances.

There is a definite correlation between the ability to hit a baseball and ocular motility. Individuals who demonstrate superior ocular motility skills have the highest batting averages. People with poor tracking abilities will have difficulty hitting a fast pitched baseball.

A device called a Saccadic Fixator can be used to sharpen reaction time and improve rapid eye movements. A board is studded with red lights which flash at random. When a light flashes, the athlete punches it and this turns it off. The more lights that are punched off in a given period of time, the higher the score.

The Saccadic Fixator is an excellent device for such sports as boxing and baseball where rapid hand speed is essential. A superior athlete may be able to punch 40 lights in half a minute while an average athlete might be able to punch only 25 lights in half a minute. With practice, scores can improve and this relates to improved reaction time in certain sports.

Another area where the athlete has superior skills is peripheral vision. Athletes have larger visual fields and react faster to a stimulus presented in the peripheral field compared to non-athletes. Poor peripheral awareness is a tremendous drawback for sports such as basketball. A basketball player must be aware of other players, both his teammates and opponents, as well as the boundaries of the court. Knowing when to stop and shoot or pass the ball to an open player is peripheral awareness.

Peripheral vision is also important in tennis. When playing doubles, a tennis player must be aware of his partner's position on the court. Also, faking a shot to one side of his opponent and hitting the ball to the opposite side of the court requires peripheral awareness. The tennis player must use his peripheral vision to be aware of his opponent's position, the net and the boundaries of the court.

A peripheral field analysis can be performed using an automated peripheral field computer. The individual fixates a centrally located spot as lights are randomly flashed in the peripheral field. The subject hits a button when he notices the flashing light. A graph of the individual's peripheral field can be generated and deficient areas are noted.

Reaction time to peripheral stimuli can be increased with training, but the size of the visual field cannot be enlarged. A visual field analysis can determine if any weaknesses exist in the athlete's peripheral awareness which may help to explain performance problems.

A sports vision analysis may also include contrast sensitivity testing. The contrast sensitivity chart uses a series of thin slanted lines to discriminate visual detail. The individual must identify the direction of the lines and this determines his ability to discriminate fine detail. This is important in such sports as tennis and baseball where the athlete must be acutely aware of the ball traveling towards him. Tennis players try to discriminate the logo on the ball and baseball players watch the stitches as the ball approaches.

Exceptional athletes do very well on a contrast sensitivity chart, frequently discerning all of the directions correctly. People with poor contrast sensitivity can do very little to improve it. Contrast sensitivity involves a neurological response of the visual system and cannot be improved through vision training.

Focusing speed and speed of recognition are important visual skills for the athlete. The eye must rapidly change focus to keep pace with the visual demands of most sports. Individuals who have an accommodative dysfunction cannot adjust their focus fast enough for such sports as baseball, tennis, racquetball or pingpong.

Speed of recognition is related to focusing speed; the object is first brought into focus and then recognized. A major league baseball hitter has a fraction of a second to decide if a pitch is a fastball, a breaking ball or an off-speed pitch. A professional ballplayer must have exceptional speed of recognition and focusing skills.

In fact, an athlete's nerves, reflexes, hearing as well as visual skills are all superior to the non-athlete. His coordination among eye, brain and muscle is exceptional.

Difficulties with accommodation and speed of recognition are treatable with vision training exercises. Treatment of accommodative dysfunctions with vision therapy has a very high success rate. The sports vision specialist can easily determine if poor athletic performance is a result of an accommodative disorder. When the accommodative disorder is corrected, athletic performance should improve.

Visualization is a popular concept in sports vision. The athlete is taught to visualize a successful image of the particular athletic activity. The baseball pitcher visualizes the rotation and path of the ball as it reaches the catcher's glove. The golfer visualizes his perfect swing and imagines the ball following a perfect trajectory to the green. The tennis player visualizes his serve exploding over the net for an ace.

Visualization, generally, does not work well for fast moving activities such as hitting a baseball or a racquetball. These events are primarily a reaction response requiring rapid eye/hand coordination.

The golfer, however, can visualize his shot beforehand since he initiates the event. Visualization can take place as the golfer is taking his practice swing or lining up his shot. By "seeing" the shot beforehand, visual memory will hopefully result in a perfect swing.

Visualization works best for experienced athletes whose visual skills are already extraordinary. The visualization process simply reinforces the perfect swing or the perfect pitch. For the non-professional athlete, it is more important to work on the mechanics and correcting visual weaknesses. When the mechanics of the particular activity are well established, visualization can then help reinforce it.

An interesting point in sports vision is eye dominance. Most people have a dominant eye which processes information to the brain about 0.10 milliseconds faster than the other eye. Everyone also has a dominant hand and foot. The majority of people who are right handed are also right eye dominant. Most left handed individuals are left eye dominant.

Eye dominance can be checked by extending both arms outward away from the body and cupping the hands leaving a tiny opening in the middle. Keeping both eyes open, view a distant object through the opening between the hands. Now close one eye and then the other. The eye that maintains the object's position through the opening is the dominant eye. The eye that is used when viewing through a camera is also the dominant eye.

The dominance is called lateral when both eye and hand dominance is the same side. When the eye and hand dominance is different, right hand and left eye, for example, the dominance is called contra-lateral. Lateral dominance is ideal for such sports as archery, tennis and bowling where the dominant hand and the dominant eye are aligned.

Baseball is the classic example where contra-lateral dominance is preferred. A right handed batter has his left eye facing the pitcher and a left handed batter has his right eye facing the pitcher.

A right handed hitter who is left eye dominant and a left handed hitter who is right eye dominant will have an advantage over a player who has lateral dominance. Indeed, studies have shown that successful baseball hitters are more likely to have contra-lateral dominance (cross-dominance).

The next best situation to cross-dominance for baseball hitters is using both eyes equally. The least desirable situation is lateral dominance since the dominant eye will not be facing the pitcher. Successful switch hitters probably have equal dominance.

Visual memory is important in the learning of an athletic skill. Positive results should be reinforced and negative results should be used as a learning experience. The greater the amount of past experience, the more information is stored in visual memory. The type of stance, the delivery, and the follow through are all a result of stored information. The seasoned athlete draws on this information and involuntarily repeats successful motions because they are second nature to him.

A professional golfer does not analyze every aspect of his golf swing. His swing is not a series of motions but rather one fluid, rhythmic motion which developed from countless repetitions. The feedback from visual memory makes this possible.

A final note concerns color perception. Colored balls have been used with varying degrees of success in tennis, baseball and golf. The purpose of the colored ball is to increase the contrast between the ball and the background allowing for easier viewing. Colored balls have not been particularly successful in baseball, but they are frequently used in golf and tennis.

Golf balls are either white, yellow or orange. Orange and yellow balls appear to be easier to spot when the ball is located in the rough. They also offer better contrast on cloudy days than white balls. Colored balls are also easier to follow in flight. The colored balls may be easier to track and locate (under the proper conditions), but they will not do anything to help improve the golfer's score. Since the golfer strikes a non-moving target and has his eye on the ball throughout the swing, contrast with the background is not important.

With tennis, however, yellow balls moving against a contrasting background can enhance the visual response and improve the player's reaction time.

Enhancing Visual Performance

Vision training for athletes can be performed in the specialist's office, a specific location provided by a sports team or a sports clinic. When the training is provided in a private office, it is usually an individual player (such as a golfer) who is seeking help. The non-professional athlete often takes this route.

Vision training therapy and exercises can also be performed in a location provided by a sports team. This method is often used by professional sports teams. The Kansas City Royals baseball team, for example, has a specific site where sports vision activities are performed.

YOUR EYES!

The final way that athletic performance can be enhanced is through a sports clinic. The Vision Testing and Performance Lab at the Olympic Training Center in Colorado Springs, Colorado, is an example of a sports clinic. The center contains sophisticated testing and training equipment. The performance level of super athletes is monitored and any weaknesses are detected and corrected, if possible.

There are various techniques that can be used by the non-professional to enhance athletic performance. Although an individual may benefit from vision therapy, these techniques can be used on the playing field to enhance performance. They are best learned during the athletic event itself.

The first technique is learning to concentrate visually on one thing at a time. When a hitter is facing a pitched ball, he should see just the rotation of the ball and not be deceived by the pitcher's arm motion. Pitchers frequently use deceptive arm motions to confuse hitters. As the ball is delivered, the hitter should not be concerned with his stance, how his hands are positioned or what type of pitch the pitcher will throw. His visual concentration should be focused only on the pitched ball.

Similarly, the pitcher should only be focused on the catcher's target. The smaller the target, the more accurate the performance. Smaller targets result in greater visual concentration. The tennis player should concentrate on the ball hitting the very center of the racket. The basketball player should pick a small target on the back of the rim and aim at this spot. The golfer should pick a small spot on the ball rather than the whole ball.

The head must be kept steady in order to keep the eyes on the ball. Uncontrolled head movements cause the eyes to stray and this reduces visual concentration. The eyes must lead the body. Football receivers should follow the ball all the way to their hands. For this to be successful, the head must remain relatively still.

Resisting eye movements by holding the head steady is also important in other sports such as golf and tennis. One of the basic lessons in golf is to hold your head still throughout the backswing and downswing and keep your eye on the ball. It is difficult to keep your eye on the ball if the head does not remain steady. During the backswing, the golfer will feel resistance to keeping the head steady. The head will have a tendency to drift back towards the club. The golfer should resist this and concentrate on keeping his head steady and his vision focused on the ball.

During the downswing, some golfers also have a tendency to pull off the ball too soon. This breaks the visual concentration and often results in topping the ball or missing it completely.

Another technique which may enhance athletic performance is watching the ball after the hit or catch is made. The football receiver watches the laces as the ball settles in his hands. Tennis players can watch the ball flatten as it strikes the racket. Baseball players can visualize the bat meeting the ball. This technique increases visual concentration and allows the athlete to focus completely on the situation at hand.

Home Exercises

Some visual training exercises can be performed at home. The exercises work best when they are designed for a specific sport. Like any exercise program, performance will not improve immediately. The proper technique and successful repetition of the exercises are required before results can be seen.

Hand/eye coordination can be improved with the following exercise. Hang a string from the ceiling and attach a tennis ball to the other end. Using a narrow stick, such as a broom handle, bounce the suspended ball off a wall. Try to keep the movement fluid and continuous. To make the exercise more challenging, use a smaller ball. This technique can improve hand/eye coordination for such sports as racquetball, tennis and baseball.

Peripheral awareness is important for tennis and particularly basketball. This can be improved with the following exercise. While staring straight ahead at an object across the room, try to name the objects in the peripheral field. Try to notice the details of objects in the periphery.

Speed and accuracy of focusing is important in golf, tennis and baseball. The accommodative system can be exercised by rapidly alternating the focus from reading material to a distant object. The exercise should be performed with one eye closed.

Before starting any vision training program, it is best to have a comprehensive eye examination to determine areas of weakness. The sports vision specialist can then help design an individualized vision training program.

Contact Lenses for Sports

The main advantages of contact lenses for athletes include better peripheral vision and comfort. Eyeglasses have a tendency to slip down the face, become dirty or wet and may distort peripheral vision.

Soft contact lenses are the ideal choice for most sports. Hard or gas permeable lenses, although offering better vision, may slip or fall out. A hard lens is also more likely to get foreign bodies underneath it, such as dust particles.

It is even possible to wear soft lenses while swimming although some precautions should be taken. The eyes should be held tightly shut when intense impact with the water is anticipated. The soft lenses may be fit larger and tighter to help prevent loss during swimming.

It should be noted, however, that some swimmers lose contacts very easily when swimming and the chemicals in the water can also cause an eye irritation in contact lens wearers. There is also an increased chance of developing an eye infection in swimmers who wear contact lenses. The issue of contacts for swimming is controversial and should be addressed on an individual basis.

Contact lenses do not offer any eye protection and protective eyewear or tinted lenses may be required. Sunglasses may be necessary for outdoor activities and are worn over the contacts to reduce glare and absorb ultraviolet light. Athletes should also keep a spare pair of contacts handy in case a lens is lost or tears during the athletic event. A specialist must decide the type of contact lenses required and will determine if lenses can be used for a particular sport.

The Need for Eye Protection

An important aspect of sports vision is proper eye protection. An incredible number of eye injuries are the result of either improper eyewear or no eyewear at all. Statistics show that baseball accounts for the greatest number of injuries followed by basketball, racquetball and football.

The greatest number of baseball injuries occur in pre-teenagers and the greatest number of basketball injuries occur in teenagers. The most serious eye injuries occur in boxing, hockey and racquetball. Data was collected by the U.S. Consumer Safety Product Commission.

Hockey injuries are usually caused by the player's sticks rather than the puck. Facial masks are the only way to protect the eyes in a fast moving game like hockey. Mandatory eye protection has been proposed for hockey players as the only method of preventing serious eye injuries.

Recently, most of the attention concerning eye protection in sports has centered around racquetball. Eye injuries from racquetball can be very serious because of the ball speed and short reaction time. Nowadays, it is **highly** recommended that all racquetball players wear protective eyeguards with polycarbonate lenses. Eyewear without lenses is extremely dangerous. The racquetball can pass through the narrow opening of lensless eyeguards because of the tremendous ball speed and inflict a serious eye injury.

Common sense goes a long way in preventing eye injuries. Tennis players should be careful when charging the net and a tennis player playing a doubles match should not look back at his partner just as he is serving. In any sport, a player should always be aware of the players around him especially in sports where a racquet or a stick is used.

Many players are injured during the warm-up period. A number of balls may be flying around carelessly and players are usually not concentrating intently. Racquetball players should also be careful when playing balls coming at them from unusual directions.

There are three basic types of eyewear protection: eyeguards with lenses, eyeguards without lenses and face shields. Eyeguards with lenses can include any type of frame and can be made with or without prescription lenses. The frame and the lenses can be molded as a single unit or the lenses can be inserted into the frame.

Eyeguards without lenses are generally useless. If the opening is too wide, a ball can squeeze through and cause an injury. If the opening is too narrow, it usually distorts peripheral vision. Eyeguards without lenses are still on the market but are not practical for any sport and may be dangerous.

Face shields or face masks are used by hockey goaltenders and baseball catchers. They generally cover the full face with comfort and visibility often sacrificed for protection. The face covering can be either wire or a polycarbonate shield.

Polycarbonate lenses are the strongest lens material made today. They are practically shatterproof and are much safer than standard plastic or glass lenses. Studies have been performed where pellets are fired at a polycarbonate lens, a standard plastic lens (CR 39) and a glass lens all of equal thickness. The glass and standard plastic lenses shatter but the polycarbonate lens repels the pellet.

All sports eyewear should have polycarbonate lenses inserted into safety frames which, ideally, are hingeless. The frame should be either polycarbonate or polamide to insure maximum safety.

At times, some athletes believe that eye protection devices hinder their performance. The eyewear may slide down, lenses may steam up or the frame may distort peripheral vision. It is true that, in some cases, eye protection devices can limit peripheral awareness. But in most cases, it is simply a question of the participant getting accustomed to the device. Players who normally wear glasses adapt quicker.

Most athletes adapt very nicely to protective eyewear and simply treat the device as part of their equipment.

Lens Tints and Filters

Certain tints and filters can be used on lenses for specific activities to help enhance vision and comfort. For example, polarizing lenses are ideal for boaters and fishermen. The polarizing process almost completely eliminates annoying glare from the surface of the water.

Mountain climbers do best with ultraviolet filters and dark tints. Actually, anyone who spends a lot of time outdoors would benefit from an ultraviolet filter in their lenses. Skiers also do well with polarization and very dark tints, preferably orange-red or grey.

Shooters find yellow or amber tints very comfortable. The yellow tint increases the contrast between the target and the background, particularly in hazy light.

II. Environmental Eyecare

The study and management of environmental factors which affect the health and performance of the individual is called environmental eyecare. The major concern is the protection of vision in the home and particularly the workplace.

Sports Vision and Environmental Eyecare

About 60% of workers who suffer eye injuries are not wearing protective eyewear. Most of those wearing protection who sustained an injury had the wrong type of protective eyewear. The National Society to Prevent Blindness estimates that over 100,000 industrial workers miss work annually because of vision related injuries. Most of the injuries are preventable by simply wearing the correct type of protective eyewear.

Certain industries are more susceptible to eye injuries, most notably manufacturing and construction. The Bureau of Labor Statistics reports that about 50% of occupational eye injuries occur in the manufacturing industry. About 20% occur in the construction industry.

Most of the eye injuries are a result of foreign bodies causing corneal abrasions. Flying particles, some the size of a pinhead, can penetrate the eye from grinding, cutting or chipping machinery.

Another common cause of eye injuries is corrosive liquids splashing into the eye. The liquids frequently cause chemical burns and scar ocular tissue. A different type of burn encountered on the job is a radiation burn such as Welder's flash. Burn injuries are extremely painful.

There are specific types of protection for the working environment. When handling or mixing chemicals, full face shields are required. When pouring furnace metal, the worker must use a full face shield composed of aluminized green acetate.

If chipping, grinding or sanding is being done, either a full face shield or cover goggles are required. Gas/oxygen cutting requires Burner's goggles. Soldering requires goggles with tinted lenses.

When performing abrasive blasting, the worker must be positioned under a blasting hood. It is usually not necessary to wear protective eyewear when under the blasting hood. Welders must, of course, wear a welding shield. And finally, machinery operation (drill press, lathe, etc.) should only be performed while wearing a full face shield.

Newport News Shipbuilding in Virginia has dramatically reduced the number of occupational eye injuries by introducing mandatory protective eyewear in the early eighties. Specific rules and guidelines were established and employees not complying with the safety regulations were severely disciplined.

In the first year of the program, eye injuries decreased by 63%. After several more years, the number of injuries decreased by 98% despite the fact that the workforce had increased.

Occupational Safety and Health Act (OSHA)

The Occupational Safety and Health Act (OSHA) was enacted by Congress in 1970 to ensure healthful working conditions. Its goal is to protect the environment, consumers and employees. The law allows for the participation of workers in safety and health matters and also establishes standards for the workplace.

The responsibilities of OSHA are the following:

- develop safety and health programs for the workplace
- maintain a record keeping system to keep track of job related injuries
- develop mandatory safety standards
- inspect the workplace and issue citations or penalties for safety violations

Inspections are conducted during working hours and no advance notice is given. After the inspection, a report is written by the inspector. Penalties can reach up to $10,000 for willful and dangerous violations. If the situation warrants it, the industry can be closed down.

It is the employer's responsibility to become familiar with the standards of OSHA. The employer must ensure that their employees use protective equipment. The employees must also keep records of workplace incidents.

Consumer Products and Eye Safety

The National Electronic Injury Surveillance System (NEISS) regulates the safety of consumer products. NEISS monitors the emergency rooms of selected hospitals to help determine the safety of products currently on the market.

The consumer product responsible for the most eye injuries is contact lenses. Hard and soft lenses cause about the same number of injuries. After contact lenses, welding equipment, batteries and power tools (chain saws, buffers, etc.) account for the greatest number of eye injuries. Some other household products that can cause eye injuries are the following: bleach, ammonia, cigarettes, paints and varnishes, glue, pens and pencils and toys.

Many injuries occur in young children. The injuries decrease as the children get older and increase again during the teen years. In fact, there is a dramatic rise in the number of injuries during the teen years.

The breakdown of eye injuries based on data from NEISS is as follows:

- Personal use   about 30%
- Home and family   about 20%
- Workshop   about 20%
- Sports   about 15%
- Home Structures   about 10%
- Home furnishings   about 5%

Vision and Automobile Safety

Many features on automobiles today are designed to help improve visibility. With poor visibility, reaction and stopping time are decreased.

Driving under conditions of fog can decrease visibility to a dangerous level. Turning on the high beam makes driving in fog even more difficult. Fog has suspended particles and using the high beam in fog causes increased glare.

Fog lights on cars are designed to point ahead and downward. The further the fog light is from the driver's eye, the more effective it is. Fog lights on cars with very long hoods are, thus, more productive. Drivers should not drive with their fog lights on if there is no fog. The lights are very blinding to oncoming traffic and serve no useful purpose.

Another car safety feature is a brake light on the back window. A study was done demonstrating a faster stopping time by the car behind when a center back window brake light operates in conjunction with the normal brake lights. As a result, all cars made after 1986 now have a center back window brake light. The result is fewer accidents, injuries and property damage.

Tinted windshields are becoming very popular. A typical tinted windshield has a 10 to 15% tint. Studies have shown that a tint this weak does practically nothing to reduce light and may be a hindrance during night time driving. The tint blocks too little sun and does not reduce the amount of heat entering the car. Furthermore, a tinted windshield will not reduce glare from car headlights at night.

Various vision tests are used by states in their licensing program. A typical vision test might include static acuity, visual fields, depth perception and color vision.

YOUR EYES!

A driver with 20/20 vision has about 4 seconds to recognize a 6 foot high object when the weather is clear. On the other hand, a driver with 20/40 vision has only about 2 seconds to recognize the same object under the same conditions. The 20/40 driver needs a faster reaction time.

Very sharp visual acuity is not actually necessary when driving. Extremely good vision is not needed when viewing large objects such as other cars or people. Dynamic visual acuity would be a better indicator of driving ability since it assesses how well a person sees moving objects.

A typical state's standard for driving a car would be as follows:

- a person with 20/40 visual acuity or better may drive without corrective lenses
- if the visual acuity is less than 20/40, the person must wear corrective lenses while driving
- a person with **best corrected** combined vision between 20/50 and 20/60 may only drive during daylight hours
- a person with **best corrected** combined vision of 20/70 or less cannot drive under any circumstances
- a person must have a combined visual field of at least 140 degrees in the horizontal direction, except the normal blind spots
- a person who has adequate sight in only one eye and meets the above requirements may drive
- correction through the use of telescopic lenses is not acceptable

If the above requirements (or similar requirements) are not met, it is the eye doctor's responsibility to inform the patient and, if necessary, report the findings to the state. Restricting a person's driving privileges is not an easy task for the eye doctor, but at times it has to be done for the safety of the driver and others.

Vision and Video Display Terminals (VDT's)

The number of people who use VDT's for either work and/or recreation has increased tremendously in recent years. The number of visual complaints associated with computer terminals has also increased. Typical symptoms of VDT discomfort include the following: headaches, blurred vision, diplopia (double vision), burning eyes and eye fatigue.

Glare, poor lighting, untreated visual conditions and faulty workstations can all contribute to the visual discomfort.

Any amount of prolonged near work can cause eyestrain. The eyes are most efficient when viewing distant objects. VDT use, however, requires concentration on a near object, usually for long periods.

It is important for the VDT operator to take breaks while on the terminal. It is recommended that a 15 minute break be taken every 2 hours. Also, every few minutes, the operator should shift his viewing to a distant object for a few seconds. He or she can look at a clock on the wall across the room, for example. This breaks the near focus and relaxes the eyes.

Proper lighting and avoidance of glare is also important. Room lighting should be half the level used in most offices. The screen should be about three times brighter than the room light. It is also best to have a sharp contrast between the screen background and the characters on the screen. These are the current recommendations by the American Optometric Association.

Glare should be reduced by avoiding open windows and other bright light sources. Window shades may be necessary to block out excess sunlight.

The workstation may have to be adjusted for comfortable viewing. Adjustable chairs should be used and set at the proper angle. The screen should sit about 20 inches from the eyes and just below eye level.

The VDT equipment, ideally, should tilt and have both contrast and brightness controls for the screen. Copy material should be kept close to the screen and within the same viewing distance to minimize head movements.

Very often, eyeglasses are prescribed for VDT use to relieve eyestrain and allow more comfortable viewing. Sometimes a pale tint is used to help reduce glare. If the characters on the screen are green, a pink tint is often used. If the characters are black, a grey tint is used.

Sometimes, a near prescription is given designed strictly for use at the computer terminal. The correction allows focusing beyond the normal reading distance. Bifocals are not ideal for computer use since the bifocal is set primarily for the reading distance. The best type of multifocal for computer use is the progressive bifocal. With a progressive, since the power changes gradually from top to bottom, all viewing distances can be brought into focus with a slight head tilt. This is ideal for use with video display terminals.

YOUR EYES!

Eye Protection in the Dental Office

The two major types of ocular damage that can occur in a dental office are mechanical trauma and radiation exposure. High speed dental instruments can project silver or tooth particles at great speeds. The particles can be projected toward the eyes of the dentist or the technician.

Radiation exposure can also affect the dentist and the technician. Soldering of orthodontic devices and blue light from curing units used to harden resins both contribute enough radiation in the dental office to warrant protection.

All of the clinical personnel in the dental office should use protective eyewear, preferably polycarbonate lenses. Individuals doing soldering should use eyewear which filters out both infrared and ultraviolet radiation. Technicians using blue light curing units should wear tinted lenses which also block out ultraviolet radiation. They should also never look directly at the light.

Patients should also be protected. If they normally wear eyeglasses, they should be permitted to wear them when in the chair. Patients should also be shielded from exposure to radiation as well.

Common Eye Emergencies

Serious eye injuries can result from chemical burns, mechanical trauma or radiation trauma. Any chemical which splashes into the eye must be flushed out immediately with copious amounts of water. It makes no difference what the chemical is, the first step is diluting the substance as quickly as possible with water. Chemical burns can either be from an acid or an alkaline substance.

Damage to ocular tissue is immediate from acidic substances. It does not worsen over time. Alkaline substances, on the other hand, usually do not cause maximum damage until 24 hours after the injury. Alkaline substances include Drano and Saniflush.

Mechanical trauma can be either penetrating or non-penetrating. Obviously, any object that penetrates the eye is an ocular emergency. But a non-penetrating injury, such as a contusion, can also be quite serious.

A punch in the eye can result in a contusion: swollen lids, black eye, subconjunctival hemorrhage, corneal edema and possibly blood in the anterior chamber of the eye. Blood in the anterior chamber of the eye (hyphema) is an ocular emergency and the patient is usually hospitalized. The trauma causes a tear in the iris and the iris then bleeds into the anterior chamber. The intraocular pressure may rise to dangerously high levels and the torn tissue can re-bleed at a later date.

Mechanical trauma can also cause a blowout fracture of the orbit. With a blowout fracture, the floor of the orbit is fractured and the contents of the orbit are depressed into the maxillary sinus. The eye usually sinks in and may appear lower than the other eye. The patient usually experiences double vision. If X-rays confirm the blow out fracture, surgery is indicated.

Trauma from radiation can affect the cornea, lens or retina. The most common trauma from radiation is from Welder's flash. This happens when the welder does not wear his protective glasses. The damage does not develop immediately; it usually flairs up suddenly in the middle of that night. The individual will wake up with severe pain, light sensitivity and blepharo-spasm which is a spasm of the eyelid muscles forcing the eyes closed.

Welder's flash causes corneal edema, damage to corneal tissue and the accumulation of inflammatory cells in the anterior chamber of the eye.

The eyes are anesthetized and then pressure patched until the following day. Medication for the pain is given as well as an antibiotic/steroid combination. The eyes are patched in order to allow proper healing of the cornea. Without the patching, the blinking eye will not allow the outer layer of the cornea to repair itself. Fortunately, Welder's flash usually heals completely in a few days. The antibiotic/steroid combination is continued for several days after the patches are removed.

YOUR EYES!

7

Common Eye Diseases and
Their Treatment

I. Diseases of the Eye

The amount of knowledge available on eye disease is immense. An attempt will be made to cover some of the more common eye disorders and their possible treatment. This chapter is strictly a summary on eye disease and is not intended for self diagnosis or should in any way replace medical supervision. The symptoms and appearances of many disorders are not often obvious and the diagnosis can be difficult. When the diagnosis is made, treatment is usually straightforward. The trick, obviously, is making the correct diagnosis. Also realize that there can be more than one type of treatment for any problem.

The reader may find it convenient to refer back to the chapter on anatomy of the human eye.

The Eyelids

The eyelid margin can be turned inward (entropion) causing the lashes to irritate the eye, particularly the cornea. The lower eyelid is usually involved.

Surgical correction is often necessary. For temporary relief, the skin of the lower lid can be held back with adhesive tape. Entropion is a common complaint of the elderly since the elasticity of the lids decreases with age.

The eyelid margin can also be turned outward (ectropion). When it involves the lower eyelid, tears may not drain adequately and tearing results. Scarring of the lids from burns or injuries can also cause ectropion. Surgery may be required to re-establish contact between the eyelid and the eye.

When the upper eyelid droops this is called ptosis. It can be congenital or acquired. The congenital type, apparent at birth, is usually a problem with the nerve that innervates the muscle responsible for raising the lid. It can also be from a muscle weakness itself. The acquired type of drooping lid can be from trauma or disease. Diabetes is a common cause.

Another common problem affecting eyelids is called lag ophthalmos which simply means that the eyelids do not close completely when blinking or sleeping. This exposes the cornea which can become dry and irritated. Mild cases can be treated with a lubricating ointment at bedtime and artificial tears during the day. When a person wakes up with a dry, scratchy feeling in his eyes, it is often from incomplete closure of the eyelids.

Eyelids very often become baggy from fluid retention. The puffiness can be from thyroid or kidney problems as well as premenstrual edema. A localized injury can also cause the fluid build up, in addition to the dilation of the abundant supply of blood vessels in the eyelids.

Infections and inflammations of the eyelids are quite common. Inflammation of the eyelids is called blepharitis. It may be caused by bacteria, oil secretions from the skin or localized allergic reactions. A classic allergic reaction can be from eye cosmetics; red, irritated, itchy skin around both eyes. The itching can be relieved by using cold compresses. Other hypersensitivity reactions can result from drugs or food to which the person is sensitive. The best solution to any allergic response is to remove the offending substance. Anything less is simply treating the symptoms.

If the inflammation of the eyelids is bacterial in nature, the appropriate antibiotic must be used. The most common infection is from staph germs which are present everywhere on the skin and tend to accumulate at the lid margins. This type of inflammation is often associated with oily skin. The treatment is very straightforward. Lid scrubs with a mild soap and warm water, when the face is washed, help prevent the accumulation of oil and dead skin cells from forming at the lid margins. With the eyes closed, the lids are gently scrubbed using a mild soap on a washcloth. The problem often resolves in a few weeks. Periodic lid scrubs may be needed since it is a chronic problem.

The most common eyelid inflammation is called a hordeolum (stye). A stye is an inflammation of the follicle of an eyelash or an oil gland. The cause is usually a staph infection. The initial symptom is tenderness of the eyelid. The eyelid usually swells and a lump forms over the affected area. The treatment is hot compresses applied frequently to the inflamed tissue to bring it to a head. Since the infection is deep within the tissue, topical antibiotics will not work. In severe cases, oral antibiotics may be prescribed. In cases resistant to hot compresses and oral antibiotics, puncture and drainage of the lesion is necessary. When it is opened, topical antibiotics may then be given.

I would like to end the section on disorders of the eyelids with a brief description of an uncommon, yet interesting, eyelid inflammation — or rather infestation. The fancy name is phthiriasis palebrarum which is an infestation of the eyelids by lice, usually pubic lice. The condition can occur when sanitary conditions are lacking. The eyelashes and eyebrows are affected. It is usually transmitted by sexual contact, but children can get it from contact with their mother. Examination of the lashes under magnification shows the presence of eggs and adult parasites on the base of the lashes. The condition is characterized by itching, redness and irritation of the eyelid area.

The entire body must be treated with an anti-lice agent and clothing, linens and grooming instruments should be sterilized.

The Conjunctiva

The conjunctiva is a thin mucous membrane, somewhat translucent, that covers the underside of the eyelids and the "white of the eye." The main symptoms of conjunctival problems are burning, uncomfortable eyes. Pain usually means corneal involvement, not the conjunctiva. The signs of conjunctival disease include edema (swelling) and dilated blood vessels over the white part of the eye.

Any type of irritation or allergic response can trigger conjunctival edema. Irritants blowing in the wind, fumes and sprays can all cause the conjunctiva to become swollen and inflamed. Cold compresses and removing the offending substance will reduce the swelling.

The conjunctival blood vessels are also very sensitive. They very often become dilated with blood. The resulting red eyes can be triggered by smog,

YOUR EYES!

tobacco smoke or chemical fumes. Exposure to ultraviolet light and certain drugs can also cause red eyes. Again, removing the irritant is the best treatment.

On occasion, a patient may look in the mirror and see a bright red hemorrhage over the white part of the eye. This is called a sub-conjunctival hemorrhage and its appearance often alarms patients. Actually, it looks more serious than it is. Picture a small drop of oil squeezed between two sheets of wax paper. The drop thins and spreads out giving a larger appearance. A sub-conjunctival hemorrhage is similar; a small amount of blood compressed between two thin, transparent layers of tissue. Trauma to the eye or high blood pressure can cause a sub-conjunctival hemorrhage. A severe coughing attack can also cause it.

Often the cause cannot be found. The blood resolves in several weeks and healing is unremarkable. However, never assume a red appearance is only a sub-conjunctival hemorrhage. The blood may be deeper in the eye and a much more serious problem. An eye doctor's evaluation is necessary to differentiate between the two.

The most common conjunctival problem is a conjunctivitis. A conjunctivitis is an inflammation of the conjuctiva often accompanied by a discharge from the eye. A conjunctivitis is usually classified by the cause; bacterial, viral, allergic or irritative.

A conjunctivitis from a bacterial infection usually results in very red, irritated eyes with large amounts of mucous discharge. Very often a conjunctival culture must be taken and sent to the laboratory in order to identify the bacterium. Then the appropriate antibiotic is administered. When any antibiotic is prescribed, never discontinue the drug too early. If the doctor tells you to take the medication for ten days, then take it for ten days, even if the infection appears to have resolved after four or five days. It is important that the bug be knocked out completely. You do not want an underlying infection taking hold and starting all over again.

A bacterial infection usually causes the lids to be stuck together upon awakening in the morning. Initially, irritation and tearing of one eye usually leads to redness and spreads to the other eye in two or three days. The mucous discharge increases and may be accompanied by lid edema and corneal involvement.

150

Common Eye Diseases and Their Treatment

The condition may take several weeks to resolve completely. Antibiotics, warm compresses and separate towels and wash clothes are indicated. Steroids are not given and the eyes are not patched.

A viral conjunctivitis, unlike the bacterial type, usually has very little mucous discharge. The eyes are very watery and not as red as a bacterial infection. The conjunctiva have more of a pinkish appearance. It starts with one eye and quickly spreads to the other. Usually, antibiotics are not given since the infection is not bacterial. The best treatment regimen includes cold and warm compresses and eye washes. A viral conjunctivitis is often very contagious and care must be taken not to spread it to other family members. A viral conjunctivitis usually starts out mild, progresses after a few days, then gradually gets better over the next few weeks.

If you treat a viral conjunctivitis, it goes away in two weeks and if you do not treat it, it also goes away in two weeks. The best treatment is to help alleviate the symptoms, make the patient comfortable, and wait it out.

Sometimes a virus can cause serious eye complications. The herpes virus can cause a conjunctivitis as well as infecting the cornea and the lids. A herpes conjunctivitis is more common in children than adults, generally occurring in children between six months and five years of age. The herpes infection occurs in one eye first then spreads to the fellow eye in about a week. It persists for three to four weeks and often invades the cornea resulting sometimes in scarring.

Humans are the only source of the virus and it is easily spread from human to human. Infection from the herpes virus leads to a prolonged disease requiring life-long treatment. Recurrent infection is a hallmark of the disease and gets more severe with each successive episode. Stress or a fever may trigger an attack in certain individuals.

Anti-viral drugs are given for herpes and steroids are positively contra-indicated since they increase the replication rate of the virus.

Another classification of conjunctivitis is allergic. A foreign substance (an antigen) is triggering an immune response in the eye. Dust, pollen and other airborne irritants constitute the largest group of antigens. Soaps, lotions and cosmetics can also cause an allergic conjunctivitis. Eye medications can also cause allergic responses.

The typical appearance of an allergic conjunctivitis is edema and dilated blood vessels in the conjunctiva. Tearing and itching will also be present, particularly itching. The best approach to managing an allergic conjunctivitis is avoiding the offending substance. Desensitization may also be necessary when the offending substance is airborne and obviously cannot be eliminated.

Management of an allergic conjunctivitis with drugs may also be required. Anti-histamines and steroids are usually the drugs of choice. Cold compresses will relieve the itching and generally help control the inflammation.

Another type of conjunctivitis may result from over-the-counter eye drops. Red, irritated eyes can develop with prolonged use of drugs called vasoconstrictors. These drugs are designed, paradoxically, to relieve red, irritated eyes. Overuse of these drops can result in a chronic, irritative conjunctivitis.

There is also a rebound effect. When the drops are used too frequently, the desired whitening effect cannot be achieved unless even more drops are used.

As you can see, many of the signs and symptoms overlap or may be missing altogether. Very often the appearance is not a textbook case or may have other complications involved. Self diagnosis and treatment can be dangerous because it can delay the correct diagnosis as well as the appropriate treatment.

The Cornea

The cornea is the clear tissue that forms the window in front of the eye through which the iris and black pupil are visible. The cornea has no blood vessels. It roughly overlaps the iris, the colored part of the eye.

The three main symptoms of corneal disease are halos, reduced vision and eye pain. Swelling of the corneal tissue can result in the halo effect and/or reduced vision. Anything that interferes with the visual axis can cause reduced visual acuity, such as a corneal scar or other opacity.

The outer layer of the cornea has a large supply of nerves and is quite sensitive. Defects in the outer layer of the cornea (the epithelium) can cause a range of symptoms; from a foreign body sensation to burning and tearing eyes to severe pain.

The central part of the cornea has no blood vessels and receives its oxygen from the atmosphere. Certain corneal conditions can lead to blood vessel formation in the normally transparent cornea. Usually this comes from a lack of oxygen to the cornea, sometimes seen in soft contact lens wearers. The most serious consequence of these new corneal vessels (which should not be there) is a lack of transparency and modification of the corneal tissue.

The cornea must not swell; it must stay in its relatively dehydrated state. If the cornea is deprived of oxygen, corneal edema (swelling) develops. The appearance of the cornea will be dull and hazy and the visual acuity will drop. When the situation is reversed, the cornea becomes clear again.

Inflammation of the cornea is called keratitis. It can be caused by an infection, an injury to the eye, a defect in the tear make-up, a nutritional deficiency or a hypersensitivity reaction.

Infections can be bacterial, viral or fungal. Often an infection of the cornea can result in a corneal ulcer, either in the center of the cornea or in the periphery. The eye is usually quite red and painful. The entire eye may be inflamed and tearing and reduced vision are likely. A corneal ulcer is an ocular emergency since vision loss can be fast and dramatic. When the pathogen is identified, the appropriate antibiotic regimen is started aggressively.

Fungal infections can be especially nasty. If the cornea has been injured by a tree branch or a shrub, the situation should be carefully watched since this is how fungal infections take hold.

Softening of the cornea can result from a vitamin A deficiency. The lack of vitamin A can also cause a dry eye condition and retinal problems. A mild vitamin A deficiency can be reversed with proper diet. A severe case will require vitamin A supplements.

As was mentioned earlier, herpes can affect the cornea. Vesicles can also be found on the lids and mouth. A tree branch pattern on the cornea develops (called a dendrite)in individuals who have had a primary infection. The virus persists throughout the life of the patient in nerve fibers in the eye. Various factors can precipitate an attack, triggering the dormant virus. *(Figure 7-1)*

The sensitivity of the cornea is diminished in an individual with a corneal herpes infection. It is rare that both eyes are infected at the same time. Typical symptoms include tearing, a foreign body sensation and reduced vision in the affected eye. After frequent attacks, the patient becomes aware of an impending attack even before symptoms develop.

YOUR EYES!

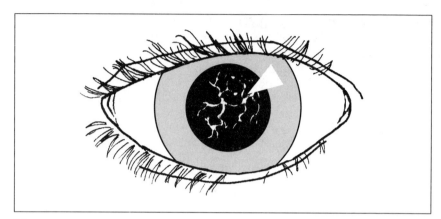

Figure 7-1 The branching pattern of a herpes infection of the cornea.

The Tear (Lacrimal) System

The lacrimal system consists of two parts; one that produces the tears and one that drains them. The secretory part consists of the lacrimal gland and other minor glands which together produce the three layers of the tears. The tears have an outer oily layer, an aqueous (water) center and a mucous inner layer. The oil layer guards against tear evaporation and the mucous layer enhances the contact between the tears and the cornea.

The tears drain through two tiny openings in each eyelid margin (called puncta) then through a narrow channel into the lacrimal sac. The tears eventually drain behind the nose into the nasolacrimal duct. *(Figure 7-2)*

Diseases of the lacrimal system can involve either the lacrimal gland or the drainage system. Tumors or inflammation of the lacrimal gland can result in swelling of the upper part of the eye, affecting tear production. More frequent are problems with the drainage apparatus. When the drainage system gets blocked, excess tearing occurs. Inflammation of the drainage system due to an infection can cause swelling and pain at the inner part of the eye, adjacent to the nose. Very often a pus discharge can be forced out of the drainage system, indicating an infection.

The following procedure is used to clear out an obstructed drainage system. Warm compresses are applied to the inflamed area followed by massaging with an upward motion to help force out the pus and mucous. The discharge is washed out of the eye and a drop of antibiotic is applied. This is usually

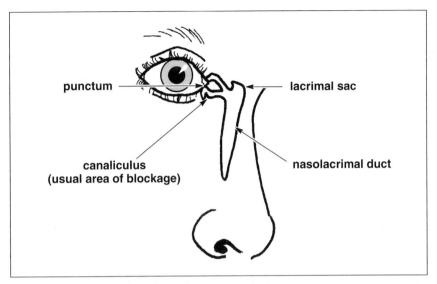

Figure 7-2 Tear drainage system of the eye. The narrow canaliculus is often the site of inflammation.

done four times a day. When the inflammation subsides, the drainage canal can be opened with a probe and an antibiotic can be used to wash the system through. As we age, the drainage passageway narrows, increasing the risk of a blockage. Usually only one side is involved and the response to treatment is excellent. Very often, infants have a blocked tear duct which usually opens up before six months. Warm compresses, massage and antibiotic drops are used. If it is not opened by six months then surgery to open it may be indicated.

One of the most common eye problems is dry eyes. This occurs when either the tear production is reduced or more common, an inadequate tear layer exists. The eyes feel dry, burn and have a constant foreign body sensation. The condition is aggravated by warmth and an environment that causes rapid tear evaporation.

Tear flow must be sufficient and of good quality. None of the three tear layers (oil, water, mucous) must be deficient. A severe dry eye problem can cause drying of the cornea and a loss of vision. Usually the problem is only one of discomfort and artificial tears used frequently can offer relief. Inadequate tears, in either quantity or quality, is the main reason some people cannot wear contact lenses.

YOUR EYES!

The Lens

The lens is a transparent, biconvex structure held in position behind the pupil by fibers. The function of the lens is to help focus light on the retina. The lens is transparent because most cells of the lens have no nuclei. A loss of this transparency is called a cataract. It is important to remember that a cataract is not a growth on the eye. It is an opacity in the lens of the eye.

A cataract or lens opacity can be present at birth or develop during the patient's lifetime. By far, the vast majority of cataracts are age-related and usually occur past the age of 50. In the Framingham, Massachusetts study, 15% of persons 52 to 85 years of age had cataracts that reduced their vision to 20/30 or less. Anywhere from 5 to 10 million persons yearly become visually disabled because of cataracts.

There are many types of cataracts. Acquired cataracts (not present at birth) can result from injury to the eye, toxic substances, systemic disease or aging. Cataracts can have various appearances, depending on the cause. Lens opacities, which are age-related, have a typical look. The center part of the lens becomes brownish orange and this is called a nuclear cataract or age-related cataract. Opacities in the outer part of the lens are called cortical cataracts and an opacity in the back of the lens is called a posterior subcapsular cataract or PSC. *(Figure 7-3)*

The severity of the cataract is usually graded subjectively by the examiner. Grade I is minimal, grades II and III are moderate and grade IV is severe. If someone has a grade IV PSC, this means they have a very dense, localized cataract in the back part of the lens.

The appearance of the cataract is not as important as the effect that it has on vision. A small cataract along the visual axis can be much more devastating than a larger one out in the periphery. The determination of when a cataract has to be removed rests solely with the patient. If the person is visually hampered by the cataract, it is time to have it taken out. The person should have difficulty performing their normal daily activities, such as reading, watching television and recognizing faces. If the opacity is not bothering the patient, surgery should be postponed until it does. Sometimes cataracts progress rapidly; sometimes they change minimally over a 20 year period.

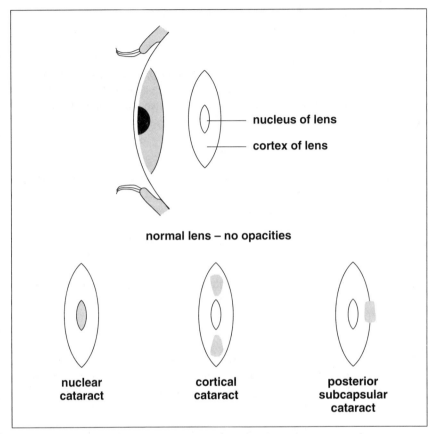

normal lens – no opacities

nucleus of lens
cortex of lens

nuclear
cataract

cortical
cataract

posterior
subcapsular
cataract

Figure 7-3 The major types of cataract.

Different people have different visual needs. A jeweler, for example, needs much more critical vision than a retired person who primarily watches television. The jeweler may opt for the surgery sooner. The important thing to remember is the decision for cataract surgery rests with the patient. Since the surgery is not an emergency, there is always time for a second opinion.

Medications can cause cataracts also. The classic example is prolonged use of steroids causing posterior subcapsular cataracts. If posterior subcapsular cataracts are noted in both eyes in a young individual, the person is probably on steroids for a systemic disorder. Since prolonged use of steroids can also cause glaucoma, persons on steroids should have a complete eye examination yearly. If any abnormalities are found, more frequent examinations may be required. The steroids may have to be temporarily discontinued or the dosage reduced.

Systemic diseases, such as diabetes, can also cause cataracts. The diabetic cataract is usually cortical, but a specific type of cataract called a snowflake cataract is a classic sign of diabetes. Snowflake cataracts are not very common, however. Diabetic patients often have an earlier onset of nuclear (age-related) cataracts and posterior subcapsular cataracts, as well.

What are the symptoms of a cataract?

The most common symptom of a developing cataract is blurred vision. Often it is most noticeable when driving a car or reading. The cataract scatters the light entering the eye and this makes focusing on the retina difficult.

Sometimes a person with a cataract sees double. This is usually when viewing a distant object such as a street sign.

The ability to judge distance (depth perception) can also be affected. Good depth perception requires the use of two eyes and since a cataract often develops in one eye at a time, most people favor the eye without the cataract. When both eyes are not being used equally, depth perception suffers.

Glare is a problem for most people but persons with cataracts are bothered more because of the scattering of light. Bright sunlight can be very irritating. Driving at night can also be very difficult because the oncoming headlights often take on a halo effect.

The distortion of colors can also be a symptom of a cataract although this is often subtle. Certain shades of blue are often distorted. This is frequently appreciated after the cataract is removed and colors once again appear bright.

Another clue to an early cataract is very frequent changes in eyeglass prescriptions. When eyeglasses can no longer give satisfactory vision to the cataract patient, surgery is indicated. Very often, however, a change in the eyeglass prescription is all that is indicated and surgery can be postponed. The simplest solution to a problem should always be tried first.

Glaucoma

Glaucoma is the most feared disease of the eye and rightfully so. About 1% of the population over age 40 has glaucoma and the incidence increases with age. About 5,000 new cases of blindness occur each year because of the disease and over a million cases remain undiagnosed. About 15% of glaucoma patients will eventually go blind.

The eye is filled with a fluid which is produced and drained at the same rate. If the fluid production is increased or the drainage system is blocked, the fluid builds up and the pressure in the eye increases. With the most common type of glaucoma, the drainage system becomes blocked and this increases the intraocular pressure. The optic nerve is very sensitive to pressure changes and the increased pressure damages the nerve resulting in visual field defects.

In the early stages, the visual field defects are subtle and are not easily detected by the patient. As the pressure stays high for many years, the optic nerve atrophies further causing massive field defects. The central vision stays intact until the very end. When the last bit of healthy nerve tissue is destroyed, the remaining vision will be snuffed out and the patient will be totally blind. Glaucoma then is high intraocular pressure causing optic nerve damage which leads to vision loss.

Glaucoma is a complex disease and can have many causes. It can result from an injury to the eye or it can be congenital. Congenital glaucoma occurs in 1 of every 10,000 births and is often associated with various syndromes. The baby usually will have large bulging eyes with cloudy corneas. The eyes will tear excessively and be sensitive to light. Surgery to relieve the pressure is the only choice.

The most common type of glaucoma is called primary open angle glaucoma and again, the drainage system becomes blocked causing a rise in intraocular pressure. By age 70, glaucoma becomes a common disease of the elderly and joins age-related macular disease and diabetes as the major causes of blindness.

The intraocular pressure can vary. It is higher in the morning than in the afternoon and is slightly higher in the winter than in the summer. It is also higher in females after menopause. Also, intraocular pressure readings can vary somewhat from visit to visit. If a borderline high pressure is detected, often the patient will be asked to return in a week for another reading.

Normal pressure values range from 10 to 21 mm Hg, depending on the instrument used. With pressure readings greater than 30 mm Hg, over 40% of patients will develop glaucoma in 5 years. With readings between 25 and 30 mm Hg, about 25% of patients will develop glaucoma in 5 years. With pressure readings less than 25 mm Hg, only about 3% of patients will develop glaucoma in 5 years.

The risk factors for high intraocular pressure include:

- smoking
- stress
- alcohol
- high blood pressure
- steroid medication

The disease is often difficult to diagnose. Some people have higher than normal pressure but have no nerve damage. Others have normal pressure but have nerve defects and subsequent vision loss. This is why simply measuring the pressure does not tell the whole story. An assessment of the optic nerve is also necessary. When the eye doctor looks in the back of the eye with his ophthalmoscope, this is one of the things he is evaluating. He is looking at the appearance of the optic nerve. With glaucoma, previously healthy tissue in the optic nerve becomes atrophied and eroded. *(Figures 7-4 and 7-5)*

As the nerve tissue erodes, characteristic field defects occur. In end stage glaucoma, massive field defects are present which spares the central vision until the very end. The person's visual field would be like looking through a straw. *(Figure 7-6)*

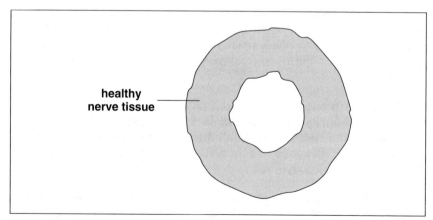

Figure 7-4 Normal optic nerve.

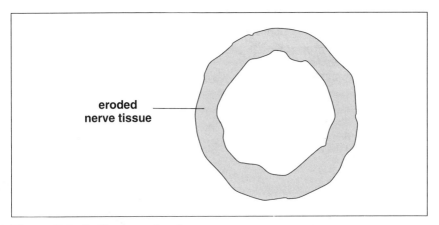

eroded
nerve tissue

Figure 7-5 Optic nerve in glaucoma.

People with diabetes, heart disease or who have a family history of glaucoma are at a higher risk as well as people who are older than 60. Also, nearsighted people with high intraocular pressure have a greater than average chance of developing visual field defects.

Nerve fiber damage is irreversible. Treatment for glaucoma is initiated to prevent further vision loss; it will do nothing to restore lost vision. Since the central vision remains intact until the very end, the patient can have massive visual field defects for years and not be aware of their condition. When the condition is finally diagnosed, effective treatment may be too late to save the remaining vision. One of the most important reasons for regular eye examinations is the early detection of glaucoma. Like most debilitating diseases, the earlier the diagnosis, the better the prognosis.

Unfortunately, even with early diagnosis and treatment, some patients will eventually go blind. Under treatment, the patient receives no feedback, warning him that his vision is deteriorating unless his intraocular pressure becomes very high. Often, the glaucoma medications are irritating and patient compliance is poor. It must be stressed to the patient that the medication must be taken continually for the rest of his life.

When topical medications (eyedrops) lose their effectiveness, the patient must be put on systemic medications which can have long term side effects. The side effects can include gastrointestinal disturbances and psychotic episodes.

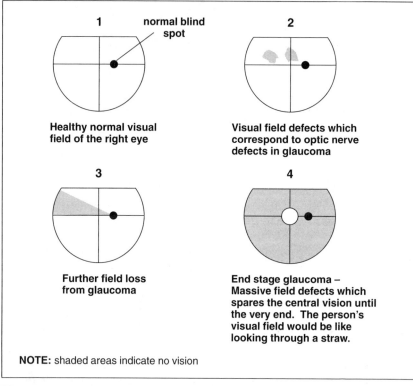

Figure 7-6 Visual field defects in glaucoma.

When systemic medications lose their efficacy, laser and/or filtration procedures are attempted. The laser treatment is called laser trabeculplasty. The laser burn scars part of the meshwork drainage system causing the remaining part to open up, increasing fluid outflow. This lowers the intraocular pressure. Filtration surgery, called trabeculectomy, also opens the drainage passageway decreasing the pressure. A trabeculectomy is usually saved as a last resort after all the other treatment modalities have lost their effectiveness.

The Retina

Age-related Macular Disease

One of the most common reasons for loss of sight in the elderly is age-related macular degeneration. The condition is also called senile macular degeneration (SMD). About half of patients seeking treatment in low vision clinics have this affliction.

Age-related macular disease will become much more prevalent in upcoming years. The U.S. Census Bureau projects that by the year 2030, there will be 65 million Americans age 65 or older compared to just 29 million today. Furthermore, in the year 2050 there will be 16 million persons 85 or older compared to only 3 million today. Since people are living longer, all age-related diseases will be more prevalent, including macular disease.

How does the disease affect vision? The macula is the part of the retina where most of the photoreceptors are located. Thus, the macula is responsible for central, sharp vision. When you look directly at an object, it is the macula that responds. Any disease of the macula will affect central vision; the most acute vision. People who stare too long at the sun during an eclipse will burn the macula.

There are two basic types of age-related macular disease, dry and wet. The dry type is from lack of nutrients reaching macular tissue due to atrophy. This process is slow and results in less severe vision loss. When the eye doctor looks at the macula, he will see clumping of pigment and other degenerative changes.

The wet type is more serious. In the healthy eye, nutrients are transported to the retina and waste products are transported away. With the wet type of macular degeneration, the transport mechanism for the waste products fails and fluid accumulates in the macula. At first, little dots of fluid are present, but eventually they coalesce to form pools. Little fragile blood vessels then grow into the pools of fluid leading eventually to hemorrhages and devastating loss of vision.

It is very important to distinguish between the wet and the dry form. The dry form has a very limited effect on vision and usually is not treated. The wet form acts quickly, often with severe results; but it is treatable. Laser treatment is administered to seal off the blood vessels and preserve vision. When laser treatment is indicated, severe vision loss occurs in only 25% of eyes treated. Without treatment, severe vision loss occurs in 60% of the cases.

The risk factors associated with age-related macular disease are:

- age, older patients are more susceptible
- cigarette smoking (in males only)

- a positive family history of the disease
- light colored eyes
- a history of heart disease or respiratory infections
- a decrease in hand grip strength

There is no cause/effect relationship between these factors and the disease. People with these risk factors, however, just have a greater chance of developing macular disease.

Individuals with light eyes are definitely more susceptible to age-related macular disease, however. These people should certainly wear sunglasses that have a UV filter. Eating a balanced diet that provides adequate vitamin A would not hurt, either. Keep in mind that preventive measures are not always successful and this again underscores the importance of regular eye health evaluations.

Retinal Detachment

A retinal detachment occurs when fluid collects between the sensory retina and the pigmented layer of the retina lifting the sensory retina away. The separation could have been initiated by a hole or tear in the retina or fluid could have accumulated without a break. The most common type of break leading to a retinal detachment is a horseshoe shaped tear which causes the vitreous gel in the eye to tug on the retina. This allows fluid to get behind the sensory retina causing the detachment.

The situation is similar to wallpaper peeling off a wall. If a hole develops in the wallpaper, it makes it easier for the paper to become loose. The retina is like a sheet of wallpaper glued against a wall. A retinal detachment is similar to that sheet peeling off.

The patient usually experiences flashing lights or floaters — a sudden shower of black dots in the peripheral field. Often it appears as if a curtain is being lowered over one eye. If the macula is affected, there will be a sudden painless loss of vision in that eye. The vision loss will remain until the retina is surgically reattached.

Retinal detachments are more common in men than women and are more common in nearsighted individuals. Very nearsighted people are at a particularly high risk. People who have had the lens in their eye removed because of a cataract are also at a high risk.

The retina must be attached as soon as possible in order to restore vision. A retinal detachment is considered a medical emergency. The hole or tear is usually sealed off and a scleral buckle is inserted around the outside of the back of the eye. The buckle forces the sensory and the pigmented layers of the retina together.

Reattachment usually restores most vision and the prognosis is generally favorable. Useful vision returns in about 6 months. When the person looks down to the ground, the buckle will be visible over the top white part of the eye. After surgery, certain activities may be restricted. Contact sports, running and jumping will probably have to be curtailed.

Retinitis Pigmentosa

Retinitis Pigmentosa (RP) is an inherited retinal degeneration characterized by loss of peripheral vision and night blindness. It is a disorder of the rods and cones — the photoreceptors of the eye. The defective night vision begins in childhood. Sometimes cataracts are also present, and if so, glare will be noted as well. As the peripheral field becomes constricted, the RP patient will be bumping into objects.

The retinal appearance will show characteristic clumps of pigment in the periphery. The optic nerve will appear yellow and waxy and the retinal blood vessels will become narrowed.

The key diagnostic test is an ERG, an electroretinalgram. An ERG measures the electrical activity of the photoreceptors. With Retinitis Pigmentosa, the activity of the cones and particularly the rods will be reduced. The rods are responsible for night vision and are located mostly in the peripheral retina. This is why loss of peripheral vision and night blindness occurs with Retinitis Pigmentosa.

The RP patient has much difficulty in bad weather and poor illumination. Traveling outdoors can be a problem. Moving from a dim to a bright environment and vice versa is also troubling.

The prognosis is generally not good. The visual field shrinks progressively over time and eventually involves the central vision. With most types of the disease, total blindness is a distinct possibility.

Gazing at the Sun

Sun gazing can literally burn a hole in the retina. The condition is called solar retinopathy and develops from gazing at the sun for longer than a minute.

The cornea and the lens absorb the sun's harmful ultraviolet rays. However, staring at the sun for more than a few seconds can overwhelm the absorptive power of the eye and burn the retina.

In the early stages, the retinal tissue swells and retinal pigment is destroyed. Several months after the sun exposure, damage to the photoreceptors develops.

After the exposure, a small, grey lesion will appear in the center of the macula. After several weeks, the lesion fades and is replaced by a tiny hole. The very center of the macula, the fovea, is responsible for sharp vision. Following sun gazing, visual acuity may drop to 20/200.

Symptoms develop a few hours after exposure. An achy feeling develops over the eyes and a central visual field defect may be present. The individual may also experience wavy vision and color vision defects.

Solar retinopathy can afflict sailors on lookout duty, sun-bathers and drug users who frequently gaze at the sun during an hallucinogenic episode. In addition, there is always an increase in the number of cases of solar retinopathy during an eclipse. Religious fanatics also frequently gaze at the sun.

Sun gazing offers no therapeutic benefit whatsoever. It can inflict serious damage to sensitive retinal tissue resulting in a severe loss of vision.

II. Systemic Disorders

Diabetes

Diabetes is a complex disorder of abnormal sugar metabolism. The hormone insulin regulates the amount of glucose (blood sugar) that is taken up by the cells of the body. When insulin is not present in sufficient amounts, glucose is not properly metabolized by cells and the blood glucose level rises causing various complications.

A normal fasting blood glucose level should be less than 115 mg/dl. Impaired glucose metabolism is indicated when fasting blood glucose levels are between 115 and 140 mg/dl. And diabetes is diagnosed when fasting blood glucose is greater than 140 mg/dl on two separate days (adapted from the National Diabetes Data Group Categorization).

There are two major types of diabetes: Type I or juvenile-onset diabetes and Type II or adult-onset diabetes. About 10% of diabetics are Type I with the onset of the disease usually before age 30. Patients with juvenile-onset diabetes must be treated with insulin for the rest of their lives.

Type II (adult-onset) diabetes has an onset after age 40 and about 85% of all people with diabetes have this type. Type II is also called non-insulin dependent diabetes. Diet and oral medications are usually sufficient to control it, although in some cases insulin may be required. Adult-onset diabetes is usually gradual in onset and the person is often overweight.

Diabetes can result in many complications. The most common cause of death in diabetics is heart disease. The prevalence of heart disease in diabetics is about three times as great as the general population. The risk of stroke and high blood pressure is also greater when diabetes is present. About 50% of diabetics will eventually develop peripheral nerve impairment. Kidney disease is common with longstanding diabetes.

Diabetes also has many profound effects on vision and eye health. Fluctuations in blood sugar can cause fluctuations in vision. Blood sugar levels should be stabilized before one has a refraction for eyeglasses. A frequent change in an eyeglass prescription is a possible indication of fluctuating blood sugar. As sugar levels fluctuate, the lens in the eye absorbs and releases water causing the vision to fluctuate.

Disease of the retinal blood vessels associated with diabetes is a major complication. Between the ages of 20 and 74, diabetes is the leading cause of new blindness. In addition, cataracts and glaucoma are more prevalent in the diabetic population.

Vision loss from diabetes usually results from retinal hemorrhages or from fluid build-up in the macular area. Sometimes, the retinal hemorrhages lead to scar tissue growth which can lead to a retinal detachment.

A person with diabetes should maintain close contact with their eye doctor as well as their internist. Medical consultations should be on a regular basis and eye examinations for the diabetic should be yearly. If retinal disease is present, more frequent examinations may be required. The proper evaluation of a diabetic patient includes a dilated examination of the retina.

Retinal complications usually occur after at least 15 years of diabetes and rarely before 10 years. After 15 years of the disease, usually some early retinal changes are taking place. When older patients are diagnosed with diabetes, the retinal changes usually occur at a faster pace and the complications are more severe.

The early stage of diabetic retinal disease consists of tiny dot hemorrhages which represent leakage of blood into retinal layers. The retinal veins often develop a distorted appearance. Instead of being reasonably straight, they look like sausage links. Often the nerve fiber layer of the retina shows micro-infarcts; the tiny vessels in this layer close down. The macular area of the retina can also build up fluid, decreasing vision.

The later stage of the disease process is something called neovascularization which is the development of new, but leaky, blood vessels in the retina. The normal retinal vessels are not functioning properly because of the diabetes and new vessels develop to try to insure proper nutrition and oxygen to the tissues. Unfortunately, these new vessels leak and the resulting hemorrhages trigger events which can lead to severe vision loss.

Recent findings, however, have shown the benefit of timely laser treatment for the fluid build-up (edema) in the macular area and for the leaky blood vessels. There are about 200, 000 people with macular edema associated with diabetes and another 200, 000 with severe vessel hemorrhaging. Another 200, 000 have both complications. All of these people are at risk for moderate or severe vision loss. Studies have shown that laser treatment can reduce the risk of severe vision loss by about 50%.

Unless the macular area is affected, the diabetic patient will have no indication of what is happening in his retina. It is, therefore, very important that diabetic patients have a complete eye health evaluation yearly regardless of how their vision appears to them.

Cardiovascular Disease

High blood pressure (hypertension) can have a profound effect on the eyes. Looking through the eye with an ophthalmoscope, the eye doctor can actually see the changes in the blood vessels that hypertension can cause. The eyes are the only part of the body where blood vessels can be viewed without surgery.

There are two aspects of hypertension which must be considered: severity and duration. When severe hypertension is present, the tiny arteries (arterioles) in the retina become narrow and constricted. This is often one of the earliest signs of high blood pressure. The permeability of the vessels eventually becomes abnormal and this leads to tiny hemorrhages, edema and lipid deposits in the retina. With very severe hypertension, the optic nerve also swells.

After many years of hypertension, the artery walls become thickened and this process is called arteriolsclerotic retinopathy. In the normal healthy retina, arteries cross over veins. With arteriolsclerosis, the artery is thickened and this causes the vein to be nicked or deflected. This can restrict the blood returning through the veins causing a vein occlusion. The retinal picture would be one of many hemorrhages because the blood backs up and leaks into the retinal tissues.

A retinal artery occlusion can be another complication. When a vein is occluded, much hemorrhaging occurs. When an artery is occluded, the blood never reaches the tissue and it dies. The most common cause of obstruction to the arterial circulation is an emboli; usually a plug of cholesterol or platelets. The emboli can come from heart tissue or the carotid arteries in the neck.

A tiny plug can temporarily block the retinal circulation causing a painless loss of vision in one eye. This is called amaurosis fugax. The vision loss can be complete but it usually lasts less than 10 minutes. People with narrowed carotid arteries often experience amaurosis fugax. Blood thinners are given because the person is at a great risk of having a stroke since the blood supply to the head is reduced.

The most severe complication of sustained hypertension is a central retinal artery occlusion. It is characterized by a profound loss of vision. The retina appears white instead of red since no blood is reaching it. It is caused by a large emboli clogging the central artery which is the main supply of blood to the retina. There will be a sudden, painless loss of vision. This is obviously a medical emergency. Retinal tissue cannot survive lack of oxygen for more than a few hours.

Emergency treatment by an eye doctor includes having the patient lie flat and applying firm ocular massage for 15 minutes. This is an attempt to lower the intraocular pressure and to increase blood flow and dislodge the emboli. Diuretics are also given to help lower the intraocular pressure. Inhalation of a mixture of 5% carbon dioxide and 95% oxygen can also be attempted. The results of treatment are, unfortunately, disappointing. A complete occlusion of the central retinal artery is rare, however.

AIDS

Acquired Immune Deficiency Syndrome or AIDS has become one of the most feared and discussed diseases of the day. AIDS is caused by a virus called the human immunodeficiency virus or HIV. The HIV virus attacks human lymphocytes which are the primary cells of the immune system. The virus destroys the immune response to an antigen, which is any type of foreign invader. The body is then left open to an attack by a host of "opportunistic" infections. Pneumocystis carinii pneumonia and Kaposi's sarcoma, a rare type of cancer, are signatures of AIDS.

The ocular complications of AIDS can include visual field defects, pupil abnormalities and eyeturns from cranial nerve involvement. Corneal diseases such as herpes simplex and herpes zoster are also found. Opportunistic retinal infections are common, cytomegalovirus (CMV), in particular. The retina will show numerous hemorrhages and signs of oxygen deprived tissue.

The front part of the eye can also show signs of the disease. The conjunctiva, the clear tissue covering the outer part of the eye, can have Kaposi's sarcoma lesions. These will appear as little purple blotches over the white part of the eye.

The HIV virus has been isolated from tears, conjunctival tissue and the cornea of infected individuals. It is unlikely that the disease can be spread through the tears since only trace amounts of the virus are found there. There has never been a documented case yet where transmission of the disease occurred through contact with an infected individual's tears. However, it has been recommended to eye care practitioners that added precautions, concerning contact lenses and instruments contacting the eye, be observed. The virus is easily killed by disinfecting agents used on instruments and contact lenses.

Toxoplasmosis

Toxoplasmosis is caused by the toxoplasma gondii parasite which can infect the central nervous system and the eye. The organism multiplies in the host cell and when the cell bursts, the organism is liberated into retinal tissue. This causes inflammation and scarring in the retina.

Toxoplasmosis is transmitted by inadequately cooked beef, cat feces or an infected mother during pregnancy. If a mother contracts toxoplasmosis during pregnancy, there is a 40% chance that the fetus will be infected. This is usually how ocular toxoplasmosis is transmitted.

The retinal inflammation tends to be present in both eyes. The symptoms include floating spots and blurred vision. The active lesion appears white in the retina and usually heals in less than 6 months. The encysted organism remains latent in the retina adjacent to the scar tissue. If vision is reduced, drug therapy is initiated.

Prevention of the infection includes avoiding uncooked meat and avoiding contact with cat feces. Women of child bearing age, who are suspect, can be tested for the presence of the organism.

Sarcoidosis

Sarcoidosis is a chronic disease affecting many systems of the body, including the eyes, lungs, lymph nodes, skin, central nervous system, heart, bones and elsewhere. It is characterized by a widespread occurrence of epithelial cell masses called granulomas. Granulomas are a type of scar tissue without cells or blood vessels.

Black Americans are affected about 10 times as often as white Americans. In about 40% of the cases, there is an ocular involvement. It is more frequent in women than men and most patients are between 20 and 40 years of age. It is most prevalent in the southeastern states.

The eye manifestations include an anterior uveitis which is an inflammation in the front part of the eye. The inflammation comes and goes. The patient will experience a dull, aching pain in the eye and be sensitive to light. There will be excessive tearing and a reduction in vision due to the inflammatory cells. Other signs include dry eye, retinal hemorrhages and granulomatous tissue, primarily in the retina.

Diagnosis is usually with a chest x-ray which will be abnormal in 80% of the cases of ocular sarcoidosis. Granulomas will be found in the lung tissue. The usual treatment for the active disease is steroids. If there is no relapse after treatment, the prognosis is good. With chronic sarcoidosis, relapse is common and the prognosis is poor.

Rubella (German Measles)

Rubella is a mild contagious disease characterized by skin eruptions beginning on the face and neck and spreading to the trunk and extremities. There is usually a mild sore throat, swollen glands and a slight fever. There can be a mild conjunctivitis.

Rubella, however, causes severe congenital defects in infants of mothers who contracted the disease in early pregnancy. There is a 50% chance of birth defects if the disease is contracted in the first month of pregnancy. There is a 22% chance of birth defects if contracted in the second month and a 6% chance of birth defects if contracted in the third month. The earlier in the pregnancy the infection occurs, the more severe are the birth defects.

There are many ocular complications in congenital rubella. These include glaucoma, strabismus (eye turns), nystagmus (jerky eye movements), retinal pigment changes and cataracts. The cataracts can be completely opaque or a pearly white opacity in the center of the lens. The retina has a salt and pepper appearance due to areas of hyper and hypopigmentation. The retinal condition does not progress.

All types of surgery are generally unsatisfactory. Prevention of rubella infection in pregnant women will prevent rubella infection of the fetus. Children are immunized with the rubella vaccine to minimize transmission during their child bearing years. Natural infection, however, offers a greater immunity than the vaccine since antibodies from a natural infection tend to be more stable.

Albinism

Albinos lack the pigment melanin in either their skin and hair, their eyes or both. Complete albinism consists of a total lack of pigment in the body including the eyes. A white person will have pale skin, blonde hair and lashes and pale blue eyes that appear pink. A black albino will be a little darker, but will have all the same features.

The albino is very sensitive to light and will usually have a high refractive error. Often high amounts of astigmatism are present. Eyeturns are common, mostly inward. Albinos cannot tan because they have no skin pigment. They often have a condition called nystagmus which, again, is a jerky repetitive eye movement.

Ocular albinism causes a deficiency in eye pigment only. The hair and skin are of normal color. Ocular albinism affects only males, but the mother's eyes will also be lacking in pigment. She will, however, have no symptoms.

Adult albinos tend to develop slowly progressive cataracts. Cataract surgery is usually advised and is quite successful. There are no field defects in albinism and the disorder is non-progressive.

The nystagmus and light sensitivity tend to diminish with age. However, the albino should guard against excessive sunlight and other bright lights by wearing protective clothing and eyewear.

The Effect of Alcohol Intake on the Eyes

Alcoholic amblyopia is a disease affecting alcoholics who are also nutritionally deficient. It only affects a small percentage of alcoholics. Amblyopia is a loss of vision not correctable by glasses or contact lenses. With alcoholic amblyopia, there is usually a painless loss of vision in both eyes occurring anywhere from a month to several years after longstanding alcohol abuse. The central vision in both eyes will be blurred and there is often a red/green color defect. The onset is gradual.

The typical alcoholic amblyopia patient is a male, between 40 and 70 years of age, who smokes and drinks heavily and has poor dietary habits. He is, in particular, lacking in the B vitamins.

Treatment is straightforward and effective. First, the dietary habits must be changed and B complex vitamins are given. Alcoholic consumption must be discontinued; often not an easy thing to accomplish. The condition is reversible if the patient gives up alcohol and establishes a balanced diet. Alcoholic amblyopia, previously thought to be rare, afflicts a substantial number of individuals since there are approximately 10 million alcoholics in the United States, with millions more considered heavy drinkers.

Myasthenia Gravis

Myasthenia gravis is a neuromuscular disorder characterized by weakness and fatigue of the voluntary muscles. It is believed to be an autoimmune disorder where a maverick antibody binds to a neurotransmitter, rendering it inactive.

The chief complaint is either double vision (diplopia) or a droopy lid (ptosis). Due to muscle weakness, mysthenia gravis patients have difficulty chewing and swallowing. They may also have breathing and speech problems and very often they cannot "pop their cheek." Emotional trauma often triggers an attack.

The disease usually afflicts young women (age 15 to 20) or older men (age 50 to 60). Females are more commonly afflicted. There are certain clues which help in the diagnosis of myasthenia gravis. When the patient blinks repeatedly, the lid droop gets more pronounced. Also, when asked to close their eyes, myasthenia gravis patients involuntarily open them a bit as if peeking. When the patient looks upward, the lid muscles quickly fatigue.

Medical and surgical intervention may be required as well as such optical devices as a lid crutch which holds the eyelid open. Eye patches or prisms may be needed to alleviate the double vision.

Hyperthyroidism

Patients with an overactive thyroid will usually have an enlarged thyroid gland (located in the neck). This is called a goiter. They will also probably have a fast pulse rate, a tremor and warm, moist skin.

An overactive thyroid can also affect the eyes. The disorder is called Grave's Ophthalmopathy. The patient will have an intense stare as if she just saw a ghost. This is due to eyelid retraction exposing more of the white of the eye. The eyes will be bulging forward, giving a frightened appearance.

They may also experience double vision due to inflammatory cells infiltrating the intraocular muscles. The eyes will be red and there will be lid edema, usually more pronounced in the morning hours.

Management of thyroid eye disease includes elevation of the head at bedtime to relieve the fluid build up in the lids. Artificial tears are given to keep the eyes lubricated and an ointment can be used at bedtime. Medical treatment consists of diuretics and steroids.

Multiple Sclerosis

Multiple sclerosis is a central nervous system disease caused by a virus that attacks the myelin sheath around the nerves. The myelin sheath nourishes and protects the nerve. The disease usually occurs between the ages of 20 and 40 and is more common in females. It is also more prevalent in cold, temperate climates.

The chief complaint is painless vision loss in one eye with occasional discomfort on eye movement. The discomfort when the eye is moved occurs because the myelin sheath of the optic nerve is inflamed due to the demyelinating disease. A common symptom of MS is a drop in vision when exercising or when overheated. Other conditions can also cause this symptom, however. Other symptoms include double vision and nystagmus. There is often a visual field defect because of the inflamed optic nerve.

The possibility of developing MS in people with immediate family members suffering from the disease is 15 times greater than for the general population. This would support either a viral or hereditary factor as a cause. There is no specific laboratory test for the diagnosis of multiple sclerosis; it is basically a diagnosis of exclusion.

There is no effective treatment for MS. Steroids are sometimes given if no vision is present or if the second eye becomes involved without the first eye recovering.

8

Medications and the Eyes

Medications and the Eyes

Drugs given for either systemic disorders or eye problems can both cause a variety of effects and complications. Systemic disorders would include cardiovascular problems, respiratory conditions, digestive conditions, etc. An example of a systemic medication would be a heart drug or a blood pressure medication.

For the purpose of this chapter, drugs will be divided into ocular drugs and systemic drugs. Ocular drugs are given for a specific eye condition and systemic drugs are given for nonocular conditions. The side effects will be divided into ocular side effects (such as blurred vision) or systemic side effects (such as nausea).

A drug works by binding to a receptor site which is usually a protein attached to a cell membrane. This interaction between a drug molecule and a receptor site alters the function of the cell. This causes a reversible biological reaction.

YOUR EYES!

Medications, like any foreign substance, can cause an allergic reaction within the body. There are two types of allergic responses, an immediate response and a delayed response.

A severe hypersensitivity reaction to a drug can cause hives, breathing difficulties and possibly even collapse of the cardiovascular system. A delayed reaction to a drug may result in fever and joint pain. In some cases, kidney damage may occur from a sustained allergic reaction.

There are numerous ways that a drug can be administered. The most convenient route is by mouth, but some drugs must be injected. Drugs that are injected must be administered into a muscle, vein or under the skin. Some drugs can also be inhaled.

After a drug is absorbed into the system, it is rapidly transported to all tissues of the body. Some cells will concentrate more of the drug than other cells. After the drug produces its pharmacological effect, it is metabolized and excreted from the body. The drug is broken down or metabolized in the liver and excreted mainly by the kidneys. Drugs can also be eliminated from the body, although to a lesser extent, by the skin, tears or expired air.

Eye medications (eye drops or ointments) can be distributed through the eye in three different ways. The medication can penetrate corneal tissue, become absorbed into the blood circulation or drain out of the eye with the tears. The tear drainage system is the usual route of drug elimination when topical medications are administered. When an eye drop is given, only a fraction of the drug exerts a pharmacological response in the eye. Most of the drug is lost with the tears.

The size of the drop is, obviously, important. The larger the drop, the greater the amount of drug reaching the eye. Most commercial droppers produce a substantially large drop to compensate for the amount lost with the tears.

The agent that the medication is dissolved in is called the vehicle. Most eye medications have vehicles of saline, alcohol or mineral oil. The rate of absorption depends on the vehicle; ointments with a mineral oil base will penetrate the eye much slower compared to a drop. Ointments are, therefore, used for conditions where a much slower delivery of the drug is desired.

For conditions of the front (anterior) part of the eye, topically applied medications, such as drops or an ointment, are usually sufficient. However, for conditions affecting the back (posterior) part of the eye, topical agents are usually supplemented with systemic medications. The drops or ointment will not sufficiently penetrate into the back of the eye.

Individuals with dark eyes usually eliminate eye medications slower than individuals with light colored eyes. The pigment in dark eyes binds the drug and slows its absorption into the body. Consequently, individuals with dark eyes may require more medication since the increased pigment binds the drug. It takes longer to build up sufficient drug levels and longer to eliminate the drug in these individuals.

The age and sex of a patient can affect how they respond to a drug. Older individuals are more likely to have drug complications, particularly if liver or kidney damage is present. The drug may not be broken down and eliminated as quickly. The very young are also more susceptible to medications.

As a rule, more adverse drug reactions and complications are reported in women than in men. This applies to both systemic and ocular medications.

The number of adverse drug reactions increases as the number of drugs being taken increases. The more drugs that are being administered, the greater the chance of a drug interaction causing a problem.

Of particular interest in the study of eye conditions is the diagnostic drug sodium fluorescein. The drug is a yellow liquid which appears green when affected areas are stained. It has a variety of diagnostic uses.

The contact lens specialist often uses sodium fluorescein when fitting hard or gas permeable contact lenses. It is used to check the fit of the lenses. It is also used for the detection of corneal lesions and to check the patency of the tear drainage system.

The most accurate method of checking the intraocular pressure is applanation tonometry. Sodium fluorescein is the dye, combined with an anesthetic, used for this procedure. Measuring the intraocular pressure is a check for possible glaucoma.

Sodium fluorescein can also be used to check for aqueous (fluid) leaks following eye surgery. The leaking fluid absorbs the dye and glows green.

Finally, the drug can be used for assessing the integrity of the retinal circulation. The sodium fluorescein is injected into a vein and rapidly spreads through the blood system. Pictures are taken of the retina through the pupil as the dye passes through the retinal circulation. This procedure is called retinal angiography and it is the retinal specialist's most important diagnostic tool. Retinal blood vessels that leak can be visualized with the use of this procedure.

How Systemic Medications Can Affect the Eyes

NOTE: all side effects listed are possible side effects; they may or may not occur. The severity of the side effects also varies considerably.

Drugs that Affect the Lids

Drug	Use	Side Effects
chloroquine	malaria	droopy lids
chlorpromazine	anti-psychotic	pigmentation spots
gold salts	arthritis	droopy lids,skin irritation
phenobarbitol	sedative	eyelid swelling

Drugs that Affect the Conjunctiva

Drug	Use	Side Effects
chlorpromazine	anti-psychotic	pigmentation spots
gold salts	arthritis	allergic conjunctivitis
marijuana		redness of conjunctival vessels
phenylbutazone	anti-inflammatory	conjunctivitis
reserpine	lowers blood pressure	redness of conjunctival vessels
salicylates		conjunctivitis, hemorrhages
sulfonamides		conjunctival scarring

Drugs that Affect the Cornea

Drug	Use	Side Effects
chloroquine	malaria	corneal deposits

Drugs that Affect the Cornea (cont'd)

chlorpromazine	anti-psychotic	corneal deposits
gold salts	arthritis	corneal deposits
indomethacin	anti-inflammatory	inflammation of corneal tissue, deposits
oral contraceptives	prevent pregnancy	edema, possible contacts lens problems
Vitamin D	Vitamin D deficiency	calcium deposits

Drugs that Blur Vision

Drug	Use	Side Effects
antihistamines	allergies	blurs distance vision
chloramphenicol	antibiotic	blurs distance vision
chloroquine	malaria	blurs near vision
chlorpromazine	anti-psychotic	blurs distance and near vision
corticosteroids (steroids)	anti-inflammatory	blurs distance vision
digitalis	regulates heart beat	blurs distance vision
diphenlhydantoin	epilepsy	blurs distance vision
diuretics	lowers blood pressure	blurs distance vision
griseofulvin	antibiotic	blurs distance vision
ibuprofen	pain	blurs distance vision (rare)
imipramine	depression	blurs distance vision and near vision
lithium	depression	blurs distance and near vision
methsuximide	anti-convulsant	blurs distance vision
oral contraceptives	prevent pregnancy	blurs distance vision
phenylbutazone	anti-inflammatory	blurs near vision

YOUR EYES!

Drugs that Blur Vision (cont'd)

sulfonamide	antibiotic	blurs distance vision
tetracycline	antibiotic	blurs distance vision
Vitamin A	Vitamin A deficiency	blurs distance vision (with overdose)

Drugs that Affect the Retina

Drug	Use	Side Effects
anticoagulants	thins blood	retinal hemorrhages
barbiturates	pain	constriction of retinal blood vessels, color vision disturbances
chloroquine	malaria	"bulls eye" pigment disturbances
corticosteroids	anti-inflammatory	color vision disturbances
digitalis	regulates heart rate	color vision defects
diuretics	lowers blood pressure	edema and hemorrhages
marijuana		color vision disturbances with long term use
oral contraceptives	prevent pregnancy	macular edema, decrease in color vision, retinal blood vessel disturbances
phenothiazines	anti-psychotic	color vision problems, night blindness
Vitamin A	Vitamin A deficiency	color vision disturbances

How Eye Medications Can Affect the Body

NOTE: all side effects listed are possible side effects; they may or may not occur. The severity of the side effects also varies considerably.

Adverse Reactions of the Eyes from Eye Medications

Drug	Use	Side Effects
phenylephrine	dilation of the eyes, alleviates red eyes	tearing, stinging, rebound red eyes, increase pressure in the eyes
proparacaine	topical anesthetic	stinging, degrades corneal epithelium, corneal edema
tropicamide, cyclopentolate	dilation of the eyes	stinging, increased sensitivity to light, increases pressure in the eyes
epinephrine	glaucoma	stinging, allergic conjunctivitis, edema in macula, pigment deposits on cornea
pilocarpine, carbachol	glaucoma	pain over the eyes, small pupils, myopia
echothiophate, physostigmine	glaucoma	stinging, pain over the eyes, myopia, cataracts
acetazolamide, methazolamide	glaucoma	transient myopia
timoptic, betaxolol	glaucoma	stinging, dry eyes, blurred vision, allergic conjunctivitis
topical corticosteroids (steroids)	anti-inflammatory	cataracts, glaucoma, decreases corneal healing, individual is more susceptible to herpes infection
idoxuridine, vidarabine	herpes infection	delays corneal healing, destroys corneal epithelium

Adverse Reactions of the Eyes from Eye Medications (cont'd)

topical antibiotics: neomycin, erythromycin, chloramphenicol, gentamicin, tobramycin		hypersensitivity reaction (irritation of tissue) most notable with neomycin

Adverse Reactions of The Body from Eye Mediations

Drug	Use	Side Effects
phenylephrine	dilation, alleviates red eyes	increases blood pressure, increases heart rate, irregular heart beat, headache
proparacaine	topical anesthetic	nervousness, headache
tropicamide cyclopentolate	dilation of the eyes	dry mouth, disorientation, hallucinations, increased heart rate
epinephrine	glaucoma	increases heart rate and blood pressure, irregular heart beat, headache
pilocarpine, carbachol	glaucoma	nausea, vomiting, salivation, slow heart beat, headache, edema in the lungs, decreasein blood pressure, diarrhea
echothiophate, physostigmine	glaucoma	breathing difficulties, nausea, vomiting, salivation, decrease in blood pressure, diarrhea, headache

Adverse Reactions of The Body from Eye Mediations (cont'd)

Acetazolamide, methazolamide	glaucoma	numbness in fingers and toes,depression, weakness, stomach irritation, decreased taste sensation, decreased kidney function
timoptic, betaxolol	glaucoma	depression, fatigue, decrease in blood pressure, irregular heart beat, breathing difficulties

Medications and Senior Citizens

Senior citizens are particularly susceptible to the effects of drugs since they are often heavily medicated. Drug interactions frequently occur from prescribed and/or over-the-counter (nonprescription) medications. Many individuals freely ingest over-the-counter medications not realizing that they may react with drugs already in their system. Some elderly patients may be on ten or more medications at the same time.

Contributing to the problem of drug interactions in the elderly is their decreased tolerance to medications. Aged individuals are more sensitive to drugs than younger individuals.

In the elderly, total body water is decreased and this allows for an increased concentration of drug in the body. Also, more of the drug is stored in fat cells and this results in a slower release of the drug from the body.

Because the cardiovascular system does not work as efficiently in the elderly, drugs are not distributed evenly throughout the body. In addition, the liver's ability to break down the drug is reduced. The kidneys also decrease their ability to excrete metabolized drugs.

Also contributing to the problem of drug reactions is the fact that many elderly patients are being treated by more than one doctor and are using more than one pharmacy. This makes keeping track of the medications more difficult. Many elderly patients have poor memories and short attention spans and this often results in confusion concerning proper dose and treatment.

Misunderstandings about proper use of medications are quite common. Some studies suggest that more than 50% of patients make at least one error concerning their drug regimen. It is very important for patients to give their complete medical and drug history when switching doctors. When several doctors are involved with the same patient, the doctors must communicate with each other. When a change in the treatment plan is initiated, every practitioner involved with the patient should be notified.

It is both the doctor's and the patient's responsibility to insure that medical instructions are completely understood. The doctor should speak slowly and clearly when explaining drug regimens. Written instructions should also be given and the patient should be questioned during follow up visits concerning proper use of their medications.

Over-the-Counter Medications

Many eye medications are available without a prescription. Most of these are soothing agents but some antibiotics and steroid ointments are now available over-the-counter. These ointments, however, should only be used under a doctor's supervision rather than the patient diagnosing his own condition.

The most popular over-the-counter drops are artificial tears. These are eyedrops used for dry eye conditions, wetting soft contact lenses and as an aid in the healing of damaged corneal tissue. The artificial tears range from watery to very oily and most people will find one or two brands to their liking. Many times, patients are encouraged to experiment with different brands in order to find the most soothing and comfortable.

For severe dry eye conditions, eye emollients may be used in conjunction with the artificial tears. An emollient is a softening or soothing agent in an ointment base. The artificial tears are used during the waking hours and the emollient is used at bedtime. Ointments are not routinely used during the day since they blur vision.

An ointment will last longer than a drop since most of the drop gets drained with the tears. Both the ointment and the drop can be applied to the inside of the lower lid. The lower lid is pulled down and the medication is applied to the sac that forms when the lower lid is pulled away from the eye. The lid is then released and the medication will reach the eye with the next blink.

Eye decongestants are also frequently purchased over-the-counter. These are drops used to lessen inflammation of ocular tissue and reduce the redness of the eyes. Eye decongestants help reduce the symptoms of allergies: watery, itchy eyes, redness and puffiness. By shrinking blood vessels, the eye decongestant lessens the body's allergic response to the offending substance. Eye decongestants should not be used to lessen the severity of an acute allergic response.

The final category of nonprescription eye solutions is an eye wash or irrigating solution. These are recommended primarily for an irritative or possibly an allergic conjunctivitis. The irrigating solution washes the offending substance from the eye and soothes irritated eye tissue.

People who work in an environment filled with dust, smoke or harsh fumes would do well keeping an eye wash handy. The eye wash is poured into the cap. With the eye held open and the head thrown back, the eyecup is placed over the eye. While looking upward, the eyes are rolled around in the head. The irrigating solution will wash the outer part of the eyeball, removing any particles or debris. This will leave the eyes feeling soothed and refreshed.

Eye washes can be used as often as needed. They will not remove the redness as effectively as eye decongestants but are safer to use on a long term basis. Concerning allergies, an eye decongestant can be used for flare ups and an eye wash can be used on a regular basis to help keep a chronic condition under control. For more severe reactions, oral medications may be required in conjunction with the eye solutions.

Contact Lens Solutions

Patients who wear contact lenses can sometimes be overwhelmed by the many types of contact lens solutions on the market today. It is best for contact lens wearers to stay with the solutions recommended by their eye care practitioner. Very often, patients develop contact lens complications as a result of switching solutions.

When evaluating contact lens problems, one of the first questions an eye doctor will ask the patient is whether a solution was switched. Patients will buy a different solution if they cannot find the recommended one or if another product is on sale. If a patient wishes to switch solutions, he or she should first contact their eye care practitioner before doing so. The doctor will know which solutions are compatible with the patient's contact lenses and which are not.

Soft contact lenses tend to become more easily contaminated than hard or gas permeable contacts. Consequently, the cleaning procedures for soft contact lenses are more involved. Soft contact lenses must first be cleaned with a daily cleaner (or weekly cleaner for extended wear lenses), rinsed and then disinfected.

There are two methods of soft contact lens disinfection, heat and chemical. With heat disinfection, after cleaning with a daily cleaner and rinsing with saline, the lenses are stored in a heater overnight. After several hours, the heat kills enough germs leaving the lenses in a sterile environment.

With a chemical cold system of disinfection, the lenses are also cleaned and rinsed. However, instead of heating the lenses overnight, the lenses are stored in a disinfecting solution. After several hours, or only minutes with some systems, the disinfecting solution kills enough germs rendering the lenses sterile.

Some disinfecting systems are purely chemical and others use hydrogen peroxide as the disinfecting agent. The hydrogen peroxide systems must also undergo neutralization. Some individuals experience burning eyes with a hydrogen peroxide system, but with proper use this is minimal. The burning is a result of improper neutralization of the hydrogen peroxide.

Some of the non-hydrogen peroxide disinfecting systems are so mild, they can be applied directly to the eye without causing a problem. These mild disinfecting solutions are often used as the rinse as well as the disinfecting solution.

There are advantages and disadvantages of cold systems as well as heat systems. Heat systems frequently break down, are bulky and require electricity. In addition, some contact lens materials cannot be heated. A few studies suggest, however, that the heater kills certain organisms more efficiently than a cold system does.

The main disadvantage of a cold disinfecting system is the cost of the replacement solutions. The disinfecting solution, in particular, can be quite expensive. Another problem is patient sensitivity to some disinfecting solutions. However, most chemical (cold) systems are easy to use and are reliable with very few problems. This is assuming patients understand the instructions and comply accordingly.

Soft contact lenses must also be cleaned with a weekly protein remover which is usually an enzyme. Protein deposits come from the tears and can coat the lenses resulting in decreased comfort and vision. With proper weekly protein removal, the lenses will remain comfortable and last longer.

The market is saturated with various types of disinfecting solutions, daily cleaners, saline rinses and protein removers. Not all of the solutions, cleaners, etc., are compatible with all types of soft contacts. Some solutions will turn certain contact lens materials yellow or brown.

Many patients are sensitive to some preservatives in the solutions. The major offender is thimerisol which can cause burning, red irritated eyes in susceptible individuals. Many salines on the market today have no preservatives and are labeled "for sensitive eyes." Even for nonsusceptible individuals, it is a good idea to use saline designed for sensitive eyes. Many patients find these salines more comfortable.

The final type of soft contact lens solution available is the soothing drop or comfort drop. These are designed for use in the eye while wearing contact lenses. The drops rehydrate the contact lenses, retard deposit formation and supplement the patient's normal tear flow. Many patients with a dry eye condition must use soothing drops (artificial tears) to help maintain the tear flow. The drops are used as needed and can be applied as often as desired.

Hard (PMMA) and gas permeable contact lenses require the least care. PMMA, the old type of rigid lens, simply has to be stored in an overnight solution. A cleaner should be used occasionally. Gas permeable contacts are similar to soft lenses in that they must be cleaned with a daily cleaner before being stored in an overnight solution. The overnight solution is called the soaking solution. This solution is also used for wetting the lens prior to insertion.

Protein removers for gas permeable lenses are sometimes necessary. Certain gas permeable materials attract protein deposits which must be enzymatically removed similar to soft lenses. Finally, soothing drops for PMMA and gas permeable lenses are also available. These drops can be applied directly to the eye as often as necessary.

YOUR EYES!

9

Surgery on the Eyes

Cataract Surgery

The most common eye surgery performed today is cataract surgery. Because of the aging of the population, the number of cataract operations performed is expected to increase yearly. Senior citizens are remaining productive and enjoying life longer. Surgical techniques have improved tremendously in the past few years. All of these factors are contributing to the increased interest in improving vision through cataract removal.

A cataract is an opacity or discoloration of the lens in the eye. It reduces the amount of light reaching the retina. Visual acuity, depth perception, the visual field and color perception may all be affected by a cataract. The patient's lens is removed and an intraocular implant is inserted in place of the old lens.

The decision for cataract surgery must be a joint venture between the patient and the surgeon. If the patient cannot perform his normal,daily activities, surgery is indicated. The question of visual comfort rests solely with the patient.

The surgeon will consider the patient's life expectancy, mental well being and overall health before considering surgery. Heart, lung or kidney disease may be limiting factors. The patient must be healthy enough to tolerate the surgery and the subsequent medications.

The patient's history is also important when considering surgery. This includes previous eye disease or injury as well as current medications. Previous surgery on the other eye gives valuable information since any complication of earlier surgery may develop again in the other eye.

The patient's vocational needs are also considered. The visual requirements of individuals are not all the same. A truck driver would need sharp distance vision under all driving conditions. On the other hand, a retired patient might be happy if he could just read his daily newspaper.

The surgeon will also evaluate the health of the eye. He may perform an electroretinogram to evaluate the health of the retina. He will also use ultrasounds to evaluate the health of the eye and take accurate measurements of the length of the eye. These measurements are important for calculation of the intraocular lens power.

If retinal or corneal disease is significantly reducing vision, surgery should not be attempted. Cataract surgery should only be attempted when a significant improvement in vision can be expected. If severe macular degeneration is present, for example, removing the lens will do nothing to restore lost vision.

The preoperative medications include drugs to lower the intraocular pressure and tranquilizers to relax the patient. Drugs will also be given to keep the pupil dilated during the operation. In patients with cataracts in both eyes, surgery is done on one eye at a time. If things go well, surgery will be performed on the other eye several months later. On rare occasions, if the patient is debilitated, surgery will be performed on both eyes during the same hospitalization.

Local anesthesia is usually preferred over general anesthesia since, with local anesthesia, the patient remains awake during the procedure.

The vast majority of cataract operations performed today are extracapsular lens extractions as opposed to intracapsular lens extractions. An extracapsular extraction removes the nucleus and leaves the cortex of the lens in place. Intracapsular extractions remove both the nucleus and the cortex of the lens. The advantage of the extracapsular technique is that it allows the placement of an intraocular implant. The implant will rest against the lens cortex.

After penetrating they eye, the surgeon will cut a hole through the front part of the capsule and, using a looped instrument, express the nucleus of the lens through the opening. Any remaining debris inside the lens is suctioned out with a tiny little vacuum like device. The intraocular lens implant is then inserted.

The eyeball is constantly irrigated throughout the surgery to prevent the cornea from drying since blinking is suppressed. The wound is eventually closed with sutures. The procedure takes under an hour and the patient is observed for several hours before being released. Cataract surgery is usually performed on an outpatient basis; no overnight stay is required.

Post operative care is very important for the next few days. As a rule, there is very little pain post-surgically. Swelling of the eyelids, a droopy upper lid and a red appearance to the eye are all normal following the surgery.

Immediately after the surgery, the eye is patched. Steroids and antibiotics are prescribed for about a week. The patient is seen by the surgeon the following day and the patch is removed. Vision is usually improved somewhat even at this early stage.

During the next several weeks, the patient must wear an eye shield when sleeping. This is to prevent any accidental injury to the eye. During the day, the patient can wear his old eyeglasses for protection.

During the next 6 to 8 weeks, the patient may be followed by the surgeon as well as the patient's optometrist. Ideally, follow-up care should be a joint venture since the optometrist will usually prescribe the patient's final eyeglass prescription as well as continuing to monitor the health of the eye.

During the recovery period, an occasional suture may have to be removed by the surgeon to help reduce the corneal astigmatism induced by the surgery.

After the eye is completely healed, usually after about two months, the final eyeglass prescription is given. It will consist of a reading prescription and usually a correction for distance viewing as well. Cataract surgery does not eliminate the need for glasses. If for some reason an implant cannot be used, the refractive power of the patient's lens must be replaced with either a contact lens or eyeglasses. The refractive power will be very high and the eyeglass lens, unfortunately, will be very thick.

Cataract surgery, when performed by a competent surgeon, is very successful with few complications. The healing process is usually unremarkable.

Occasionally, a few complications can arise. Macular edema, a fluid build up in the area of the retina responsible for sharpest vision, sometimes occurs several months following surgery. Visual acuity may drop as low as 20/200. Usually, the condition resolves after several months.

Another postoperative complication is hemorrhaging in the anterior chamber of the eye. This also usually resolves with time.

A more serious complication, although fortunately rare, is endophthalmitis: an inflammation of the intraocular tissues. The patient will experience severe pain and eyelid swelling. An infection may develop. Prompt treatment with antibiotics is essential to prevent loss of visual function.

Another serious complication following cataract surgery is a retinal detachment. Retinal detachments occur in about 1% or post-surgical cases, usually within six months. If detected early, a retinal specialist may be able to restore most lost vision by reattaching the retina.

A very common development, following extracapsular lens extraction, is the opacification of the remaining capsule of the lens. The opacification is called the "after cataract" and it is easily removed with the use of a laser. After the opacification is removed, more light will reach the retina and vision will be markedly improved.

In recent years, improvements in surgical techniques for cataract removal have been remarkable. If the patient's visual acuity is unacceptable to him and there are no contraindications to surgery, the patient should seriously consider having the operation. After the surgery, many patients remark that they should have had the operation years ago.

Glaucoma Surgery

The initial treatment plan for glaucoma is medication, either drops or medications taken by mouth. After years of treatment, glaucoma medications often lose their effectiveness. At this stage, surgery is often contemplated.

The goal of treatment, for both drugs and surgery, is lowering of the intraocular pressure. The eyeball contains a fluid which is normally produced and drained at the same rate. If the drainage system gets clogged (and the fluid is still being produced at the same rate), the fluid level rises. This increases the pressure inside the eye, called the intraocular pressure, which may cause optic nerve damage and subsequent vision loss.

One of the most important steps in an eye examination is the measurement of the intraocular pressure.

There are two basic types of glaucoma surgery: iridectomy and trabeculectomy. An iridectomy is a surgically made passageway through the iris. It can be performed with either a knife or a laser. An iridectomy is done when the drainage system of the eye is very narrow or blocked completely. The surgery creates an artificial passageway to allow drainage of the intraocular fluid. The procedure is relatively simple and requires no hospitalization.

Most iridectomies performed today are done with an argon laser, as opposed to a knife. There is less trauma to the eye and the healing process is more rapid.

A trabeculectomy is a procedure where the drainage system of the eye, called the trabecular meshwork, is enlarged. As with an iridectomy, it can be performed with either a knife or a laser. The effect of both procedures is the same; to facilitate the outflow of the fluid and subsequently reduce the pressure inside the eye.

An iridectomy is usually performed if the patient is less than 50 years of age and has a trend of rising intraocular pressure. It is also done if the drainage system is anatomically narrow or if the patient has recurrent attacks of high pressure.

A trabeculectomy is performed if marked changes in the optic nerve are noticed or if the patient is experiencing a visual field loss.

Complications of glaucoma surgery include excessive filtration, intraocular bleeding, cataracts and a sudden rise of intraocular pressure post-surgically. The sudden rise of intraocular pressure is the greatest concern since it may wipe out any remaining vision. These procedures are usually reserved for patients with end stage glaucoma who probably have very little vision remaining.

Glaucoma surgery will not restore lost vision; optic nerve damage cannot be reversed. It is used to prevent further vision loss by reducing the intraocular pressure.

Laser surgery on the trabecular meshwork is very safe but not particularly effective. On the other hand, a surgical passageway through the iris is very effective in lowering intraocular pressure but has many complications.

The decision for glaucoma surgery is not an easy one. The risks versus the benefits must be weighed very carefully. Very often, one problem is substituted for another. With end stage glaucoma, with or without surgery, the prognosis is bleak.

Retinal Detachment Surgery

Retinal detachments are more prevalent in nearsighted individuals and in patients following cataract surgery. Actually, any type of eye surgery that affects the retinal-vitreous interface increases the chance of a retinal detachment.

Nearsighted eyes are long eyes and this results in the retina becoming stretched over the back of the eye. A stretched or thinned retina is more susceptible to holes or tears.

The retina is a thin, transparent tissue attached to the inner wall of the back of the eye. A hole or tear in the retina allows fluid to leak behind the retina lifting it away from its attachment. This is a retinal detachment and it results in a sudden, dramatic, painless loss of vision. If the retina is not reattached quickly, vision will be permanently lost. A retinal detachment is a medical emergency.

The retinal specialist will carefully examine the entire retina for tiny holes or breaks. Before the reattachment surgery, all holes must be located by the surgeon in order to be sealed by cryotherapy. Cryotherapy is a freezing technique where the margins of the break are sealed down against the underlying pigment. A freezing probe is pressed against the retinal tissue.

After the breaks are sealed, a scleral buckle is inserted behind the globe and tightened against the back of the eye. The buckle forces the back of the globe forward, reattaching the retina to the back of the eye. The buckle will either encircle the entire globe or just a segment of it. The surgeon's incision will vary from 360 degrees for an encircling buckle to 180 degrees for a segmental buckle. The extraocular muscles will be strapped to the side with a suture during the procedure to keep them out of the way.

Silicone implants are placed under the buckle to permit further indentation of the globe. The implants vary in size for different degrees of indentation.

After the scleral buckle is in place, the surgeon will check the blood supply to the retina to insure that it has not been choked off by the buckle. The intraocular pressure of the eye will also be monitored carefully.

There are usually very few complications, postoperatively. After the first day, patients are ambulatory and have very little discomfort. Steroid drops may be necessary if there is any sign of inflammation following the surgery. If the cornea becomes hazy following the operation, it may be a sign of high intraocular pressure which must be addressed.

If severe pain is present in the early postoperative period, an infection may be present necessitating the use of appropriate antibiotics.

The patient may experience diplopia (double vision) following the surgery. This is because of trauma to the extraocular muscles which control eye movement. The double vision disappears in a few months. Scleral implants can induce a refractive error since they alter the shape of the globe. The encircling type of buckle usually causes an increase in nearsightedness. The buckle is a permanent fixture, thus, glasses need to be prescribed for the refractive error. The refractive error remains stable throughout life.

Retinal detachment surgery is successful over 80% of the time. Sometimes, a second operation is required. Visual acuity improves to better than 20/50 in more than 50% of patients following retinal detachment surgery. Vision may not be perfect following surgery, but diminished vision is better than no usable vision at all.

Eyelid Muscle Surgery

The eyelids provide protection for the eyes and distribute and eliminate the tears. They are covered by very thin skin and loose tissue. The muscles of the eyelid consist of the orbicularis fibers which close the lids and the levator muscle which raises the lid.

The two major types of eyelid surgery are surgical corrections for lids turning inward or outward and blepharoplasty which is cosmetic surgery for baggy or sagging lids.

An eyelid turning inward is called an entropion. It occurs frequently with advancing age and is then called senile entropion. The eyelid margin rolls inward because of spasms of the orbicularis muscle and also because the eyelid tissue becomes more loose with age. This leads to a red, watery, scratchy eye because the eyelashes turning inward irritate the cornea. Usually, just the lower lid margin rolls inward.

An eyelid turning outward is called an ectropion and also occurs primarily in the lower lid. The lid becomes everted and is not making contact with the globe. The tears cannot drain properly and stream down the patient's face. As the condition progresses, the exposed lid tissue becomes thick and irritated.

With ectropion, the sagging of the lower lid and the failure of the upper lid to close results in corneal exposure and subsequent drying of the cornea.

Both ectropion and entropion can be corrected with surgery. The tissue is tightened horizontally establishing the normal lid position with the globe. The surgery is very straightforward and the results are usually excellent.

Another type of eyelid surgery is for the correction of eyelid retraction. In most people, the upper eyelid margin rests just above the pupil. The white of the eye is not normally visible below the upper lid above the cornea.

In some conditions, most notably thyroid disease, the upper lid becomes retracted back exposing the white of the eye above the cornea. The person with retracted eyelids appears as if he has just seen a ghost. The eyes protrude and bulge forward. This is the classic sign of Grave's thyroid disease. The lids do not close properly and the cornea can become dry and irritated.

The lid retraction can be corrected surgically by lengthening the retractor muscle in the lid. The major complication postoperatively is severe lid edema which is common with thyroid disease anyway.

Blepharoplasty is the removal of excess skin folds and fat deposits from the upper and lower lids. In the older age groups, it is done to primarily correct a visual obstruction. It is usually done in the younger age groups to improve the cosmetic appearance of the patient.

The procedure does not remove skin pigmentation or deep wrinkles. Prior to the procedure, it is important to control the patient's blood pressure, and any medications that interfere with blood clotting must be avoided.

Contraindications for blepharoplasty include a dry eye condition, weak closure of the eyelids, preexisting eye disease or patients with unrealistic expectations.

After the procedure, the patient is administered steroids to reduce postoperative swelling. Crushed ice wrapped in a towel is applied for the first 24 hours. During the following two weeks, the puffiness and discomfort gradually diminishes. Furthermore, the eyelids may become stiff during the healing process, but they comfortably loosen with time.

As people become more appearance conscious, cosmetic eyelid surgery is becoming more popular. Individuals with saggy puffy eyelids, who are bothered by their appearance, should consult with a surgeon who specializes in eyelid surgery.

Surgery on the Tear (Lacrimal) Drainage System

The lacrimal system is the tear drainage system of the eye. Tears drain through tiny holes in the lid margins called puncta. The puncta drain into little channels called canaliculi which then drain into the lacrimal sac. The lacrimal sac turns into the bony nasolacrimal duct which empties behind the nose.

Often, the drainage passageway becomes blocked or, in the case of some infants, does not develop properly. With infants younger than 6 months of age, a nonsurgical approach is attempted first.

Dacryostenosis is a blockage of the nasolacrimal duct. When this occurs in infants, the area above the lacrimal sac is massaged and topical antibiotics are given to the infant by the parents. Parents will also be given instructions on lacrimal sac massage. They will place an index finger over the inner area of the lower lid and massage down and toward the nose. This will be done to hopefully free the blockage.

If this conservative treatment does not work, surgery will be attempted. A persistent blockage of the nasolacrimal passageway can lead to a serious infection of the lacrimal system.

The child will be placed under general anesthesia and the surgeon will probe the lacrimal passageway. The passageway will be widened by the probe. An irrigating solution of antibiotic and steroids may then be injected through the passageway to help clear the opening.

In some cases, a newborn may have an acute dacryocystitis which is a severe infection of the nasolacrimal duct. In this situation, the conservative approach may not be used and the lacrimal passageway will be probed before two months of age.

Various signs of inflammation may be present with an acute dacryocystitis. The infant may have a fever and a high white blood cell count which indicates a systemic infection. The area between the eye and nose will be swollen, red and extremely sensitive. Antibiotics will be needed to control the infection.

In some stubborn cases of a blocked drainage system, a narrow tube is inserted through the nasolacrimal passageway to force it open. The tubing is kept in place for up to six months before removal. If successful, the nasolacrimal duct will remain in an expanded position.

If all else fails and the nasolacrimal duct remains blocked, a dacryocystorhinostomy is performed. With this procedure, an artificial passageway is made from the nose to the drainage system. Patients must be admitted prior to surgery and are discharged the following morning.

There is very little edema following surgery. Systemic antibiotics are usually given for three days. Sometimes, a tube is inserted during the procedure and removed after six weeks. After a dacryocystorhinostomy, tears will drain freely and recurrent infections of the drainage system will no longer occur.

Sometimes, an overflow of tears may not be due to a blocked drainage system but rather a reflex response to a dry eye condition. Because the eyes are dry, the lacrimal gland produces extra tears which overwhelm the drainage system and then flow down the face.

There are several tests that the eye doctor can perform to check the patency of the drainage system. One test is called the Taste Test. Saccharine drops are added to the eye and, after a period of time, the patient should taste the drops. This shows that the nasolacrimal system is open since the passageway drains into the throat and the solution can then be tasted.

Another test is called the Jones Dye Test. With this test, a drop of dye is inserted into the eye. The nostril on the same side is sprayed with a topical anesthetic and a small wire wrapped with cotton is inserted up the nose. The cotton is removed after 5 minutes. If dye is present on the cotton, the tear drainage system is normal.

Surgery on the Cornea

The cornea is the normally transparent tissue covering the outer part of the eye. It approximately covers the colored part of the eye, the iris. The cornea contributes to the refractive state of the eye and its transparent structure permits light rays to pass unimpeded to the retina.

The cornea is the only ocular tissue that can accept a transplant. Donor corneas are stored at an eye bank which can maintain healthy corneas for about a week. At some eye banks, corneas can be stored in liquid nitrogen for months, although this procedure is difficult and expensive.

Cornea transplant surgery is called penetrating keratoplasty. It is usually done to improve visual acuity by removing an opaque or diseased cornea. Indeed, some bacterial or fungal infections can completely destroy the cornea.

The most common reason for a corneal transplant is corneal complications following a cataract removal. The cornea becomes swollen and non-functioning following surgery to remove the lens. Other indications for a corneal transplant include perforations of the cornea, dense corneal scars or degenerative disorders of the cornea.

The patient's visual acuity will be carefully assessed before the operation as well as his intraocular pressure. If the pressure inside the eye is high, the prognosis for a successful transplant is not good.

Preoperative medications include antibiotics and sedatives. A local anesthetic is used and the patient is discharged on the second day following the operation.

The corneal surgeon uses an instrument called a trephine for removing a circular area of the cornea. The circular blade is pressed against the cornea and rotated back and forth until it penetrates the cornea to the desired thickness. The opaque cornea is then lifted away. The donor cornea is then transferred to the eye and sutured in place. The sutures are placed radially around the cornea. *(Figure 9-1)*

Following the surgery, steroids and antibiotics are given. The eye must be protected full time for three months after corneal surgery. Eyeglasses are worn during waking hours and a metal shield is worn at bedtime.

The patient's activities must also be restricted. Heavy objects cannot be lifted and no swimming is allowed.

Topical antibiotics are used until the cornea heals completely and steroid drops are used for several weeks and then tapered. If the transplant is performed for herpes simplex corneal disease, antiviral drops must also be administered.

The sutures are removed two months after the surgery. Most patients require glasses after the surgery although some patients may have excellent

YOUR EYES!

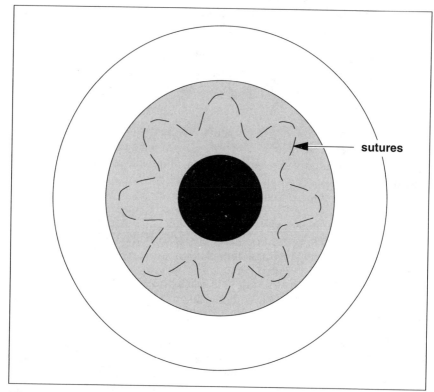

Figure 9-1 Corneal transplant.

uncorrected vision. Gas permeable contact lenses are sometimes used to correct any astigmatic refractive error induced by the surgery. Soft contact lenses cannot be used because, following corneal surgery, there is a tendency for vascularization of corneal tissue. Vascularization is abnormal blood vessel growth and this is aggravated by soft contact lenses.

If the transplanted cornea never becomes clear, this is graft failure. A transplant that does not take can result from surgical trauma or a defective donor cornea. It is possible, in fact, that the donor cornea was infected prior to transplantation. A repeat transplant can be performed, however.

A transplanted cornea that does not take is attacked by the immune system of the host. The signs of tissue rejection are decreased vision, pain, and redness. During the healing process, the patient is instructed to check his vision daily, and report any changes immediately.

Surgically induced astigmatism is the main factor limiting acuity after the procedure. The surgery causes an irregular shape to the cornea and this distorts the patient's vision.

The prognosis for keratoplasty depends on why the procedure was done. Certain corneal disorders offer a better prognosis for a successful implant. Damage to the cornea during cataract surgery offers a good prognosis, for example. On the other hand, damage to the cornea from chemical or radiation burns has a much poorer success rate.

Surgical Removal of the Vitreous Gel

Removing the vitreous gel because of eye disease is called a vitrectomy. The vitreous gel is a fluid like substance, almost all water, which fills and gives shape to the eyeball. It is located primarily behind the lens and in front of the retina.

The health of the retina and the optic nerve must be evaluated before the vitreous is removed. It would not make any sense to go through all the trouble of a vitrectomy if the retina was not functioning reasonably well.

An incision is made near the border of the cornea and a hollow needle is carefully inserted. The vitreous is sucked through the needle by an infusion device. During the procedure, an irrigating solution is injected at the same rate to substitute for the vitreous. This maintains the same intraocular volume. If this was not done, the eyeball would collapse and the retina would detach.

A vitrectomy is indicated when the vitreous gel becomes opaque due to a hemorrhage or inflammatory cells. The opaque media blocks light from reaching the retina and reduces vision.

Many surgeons prefer to wait six months after a retinal hemorrhage leaks into the vitreous before doing a vitrectomy. Very often, the blood becomes reabsorbed and vision returns. However, sometimes during the waiting period, the retina can detach because the hemorrhage in the vitreous tugs on it.

A severe complication of diabetic retinal disease is vitreous hemorrhage. Because of the diabetes, the retinal blood vessels become leaky and hemorrhage into the vitreous. Most of these patients can achieve significant improvement in their vision following a vitrectomy.

A special vitrectomy procedure is sometimes done when a patient has a large retinal tear. The retina peels off and rolls over on itself. A vitrectomy is performed and the vitreous is replaced with a gas. As the gas is injected, it rises against the retina, unfolding it. The gas is left in the eye long enough to allow the retina to reattach. When the retina is reattached, a fluid-gas exchange is done; the gas is removed and a liquid is substituted.

A vitrectomy is also done when a foreign body, such as a piece of metal, enters the interior of the eye. If the intraocular foreign body is magnetic, a giant magnet can be used to draw it out safely. If a nonmagnetic foreign body enters the vitreous, a vitrectomy is indicated.

A severe introcular inflammation, called endophthalmitis, is another indication for a vitrectomy if inflammatory cells fill the vitreal cavity. It is usually associated with an infection. A vitrectomy will remove the dead inflammatory cells as well as the bacteria. Usually, the vitrectomy is combined with antibiotic therapy injected into the vitreal cavity.

There are several complications which may arise following a vitrectomy. One of the most serious complications is neovascular glaucoma. Neovascular glaucoma is the development of blood vessels in the fluid drainage system of the eye. The intraocular fluid cannot drain properly and the pressure inside the eye rises. This is a frequent complication with diabetic patients.

Another surgical complication is corneal decompensation. The cornea is traumatized by the surgery and, in some cases, a corneal transplant is required. Corneal problems are more likely in diabetic patients too.

During a vitrectomy, a retinal tear can sometimes occur when a surgical instrument nicks the retina. The retinal tear can lead to a retinal detachment.

A final complication is recurrent hemorrhaging. Following the vitrectomy, the retinal vessels may continue to leak into the vitreous. This is a frequent problem when the patient has advanced diabetic retinal disease.

Retinal Laser Surgery

A laser is a light stimulated by radiation. A current is passed through a gas in a laser tube. A cascade of photons is generated, producing a laser beam. The power of the laser can be increased by increasing the current, and this generates more photons.

The effect of the laser on retinal tissue is thermal coagulation: heat destruction of retinal proteins. The intensity of the laser is increased by either prolonging the exposure time or increasing the power.

The advantage of laser treatment is that the heat generated by the laser remains precisely at the site of absorption. It does not spread to adjacent tissue. The diameter of the laser beam can be made quite narrow and directed to very specific areas of the retina. Laser treatment results in tiny little burn holes in the retina.

The majority of retinal laser surgery is used for the treatment of diabetic retinal disease. The process is called photocoagulation, and it is used to destroy leaking blood vessels. The laser treatment seals off the vessels. If left untreated, the leaking blood vessels hemorrhage which can compromise vision.

Another complication of diabetic retinal disease is maculopathy which is edema in the macular area of the retina. Early studies of photocoagulation for macular edema suggest only a marginal improvement in vision following treatment. Treatment is directed at areas of leakage.

A specific type of photocoagulation is called panretinal photocoagulation. With panretinal photocoagulation, the retinal specialist administers from 800 to 1600 tiny laser burns throughout the patient's retina. This treatment destroys present vessel leakage as well as preventing future vessel growth. Panretinal photocoagulation is used for severe diabetic retinopathy with decent success. The Diabetic Retinopathy Study suggests that panretinal photocoagulation can be used successfully for high risk individuals. The results show that there is a 50% reduction in severe vision loss over a two year period with treatment.

Photocoagulation of retinal tissue can be used for other disorders as well. Sickle cell anemia can lead to leaky retinal vessels, and laser photocoagulation has been attempted for this condition. The long term benefits have yet to be established.

Photocoagulation is also used for the treatment of a central retinal vein occlusion. The retinal arteries carry blood to retinal tissue and the retinal veins drain the blood from the tissue. If the central retinal vein becomes occluded, the blood supply from the retina backs up behind the occlusion. This results in massive hemorrhages throughout the retina. The hemorrhages usually reabsorb, but a complication of the disorder is leaky blood vessels. The leaky blood vessels can be successfully treated with photo-coagulation.

Argon blue-green laser treatment has also been used for senile macular de-generation, also called age-related maculopathy. The disorder is the lead-ing cause of new blindness in the United States. In advanced stages of mac-ular degeneration, blood vessels under the retina can become leaky. This is called a sub-retinal neovascular membrane.

Very tiny laser burns are administered over the leaky vessels to try to prevent further leakage. The treatment is not a cure for senile macular degeneration since it does nothing to alter the underlying disease process.

Complications of retinal laser surgery include the following: loss of vision, cataracts, corneal damage and increased interocular pressure. The corneal damage and the increased intraocular pressure are usually temporary.

Removing the Eye – Enucleation and Evisceration

The decision to remove an eye is, obviously, difficult for both patient and doc-tor. Indications for removal of an eye include severe trauma, an inoperable tumor or a blind, painful eye.

Removal of the entire globe is called enucleation and removal of just the con-tents of the eye is called evisceration.

Whenever an eye has to be removed, an evisceration is the preferred proce-dure, if possible. It is more acceptable to the patient if the entire eye is not removed. In addition, an evisceration offers a better cosmetic appearance than an enucleation. It is also an easier surgical procedure, and it does not require cutting the optic nerve.

The only advantage to an enucleation is the prevention of any spreading of an ocular tumor since the entire eye is removed.

After the eye is removed, an antibiotic/steroid ointment is inserted, and a firm pressure bandage is applied. The bandage remains for several days. There is usually minimal pain post-operatively.

Four to six weeks after the surgery, a prosthesis is fitted: an artificial eye. An impression-molded prosthesis is usually fitted by an ocularist. The patient frequently adapts very quickly to the artificial eye. Occasional use of lubri-cant eye drops is required to insure easy movement of the prosthesis.

The prosthesis can be removed and polished or refit by the ocularist.

The eye has more natural movement following evisceration as opposed to enucleation. With evisceration, the extraocular muscles remain intact. This allows for more coordinated eye movement.

YOUR EYES!

10

The Eye and Aging:
Subnormal Vision

The Eye and Aging

People are living longer and remaining active and productive in their later years. Since 1900, 26 years have been added to the average life expectancy in this country. The fastest growing age group of the American population is the over 85 group.

It is estimated that, by the year 2000, there will be about 75 million Americans age 50 or older. The number of Americans age 65 or older will total 30 million.

About 25% of the over 65 group are visually impaired. It is projected that, by the year 2000, the number of individuals over 65 with severe visual impairment will double. Visual impairment is a severe loss of usable vision, usually caused by advanced eye disease. Because the population is growing older, there is increasing interest in the normal changes of the aging eye as well as the consequences of subnormal vision.

YOUR EYES!

Normal Physical Changes of the Aging Eye

These are normal changes of the aging eye as opposed to abnormal changes caused by eye disease.

The tissue adjacent to the eye undergoes some noticeable changes as the years pass by. There is a loss of orbital fat which normally surrounds the eye in its socket. With advancing years, this gives the eyes a hollow or sunken appearance.

The surrounding tissue also loses muscle tone and elasticity. The skin tends to fold over the upper lid. This condition is called blepharochylasis and is quite common with the older age groups. The extra fold of skin can increase pressure on the eye and can also reduce overhead vision.

The aging retina undergoes dramatic changes, as well. There is a loss of photoreceptors which are responsible for converting the light energy into chemical energy. This loss affects visual processing.

The blood supply to the peripheral retina decreases as the eye ages. This may explain the loss of the peripheral field which many older adults experience. The retinal pigment also undergoes alterations; it tends to become clumped as degenerative changes occur.

The macular area of the retina often develops tiny deposits of hyaline called drusen. When looking at the retina with an ophthalmoscope, they appear as little, yellow specks dotting the posterior pole of the retina. The drusen are end products of the aging photoreceptors.

The retinal blood vessels also show the effects of aging. The retinal arteries, like the arteries everywhere in the body, become sclerosed and narrowed. This reduces the blood flow to the retina and may diminish vision.

With advancing age, the cornea loses its normal transparency. Corneal tissue becomes lackluster in appearance. The endothelial cells of the cornea, which do not regenerate, are markedly reduced in number. A reduced tear flow, resulting in the very common dry eye condition, damages the corneal epithelium.

In addition, lipid deposits accumulate in a circular pattern in the aging cornea. This is called arcus senilis and is visible as a cloudy ring encompassing the periphery of both corneas. This loss of corneal clarity can also affect the quality of vision.

The Eye and Aging: Sub-normal Vision

The lens of the eye undergoes significant age-related changes. After years of absorbing ultraviolet light, the proteins in the lens are altered. The lens develops a brownish orange appearance called brunescence. If the brunescence becomes advanced and dramatically reduces vision, it is called a nuclear cataract. Mild brunescence is a normal aging change of the lens; a cataract is a progression of this process leading to a disease state.

Another normal aging change of the lens is the appearance of occasional fluid-filled sacs in the lens cortex.

The distinction between normal brunescence and cortical changes and cataracts is vague. If the lens changes are not significantly affecting vision, they are usually just considered age-related changes.

Presbyopia is another age related change of the lens. The lens loses its ability to focus on near objects such as reading material. The lens gradually loses its near focusing ability until it is lost completely at about age 65. Reading glasses or bifocals are used to compensate for the loss of near vision.

The vitreous gel, which fills the eye, also undergoes changes as a person ages. The gel becomes more liquid-like and shrinks with age. A vitreous detachment, where the gel pulls away from the retina, is a common degenerative change and is not considered a disease process. As the vitreous undergoes liquidification, the normal cells and debris floating in the vitreous become annoying to the patient. Floating strands or "cobwebs" are a common complaint.

The aging changes of the cornea, lens and vitreous all adversely affect vision by scattering incoming light. The light is diffracted and scattered throughout the internal eye. This reduces the light transmission to the retina and compromises vision.

Still other aging changes affect the pupil. The muscles of the iris atrophy with age and this results in a sluggish pupil. In the young eye, bright light causes a rapid constriction (narrowing) of the pupil. In dim light, the pupil dilates (enlarges). This effect still occurs in elderly people but the response is slower. The pupil constricts when exposed to a bright light, but it takes longer.

Older individuals also have significantly smaller pupils. As a person ages, the pupil diameter gradually decreases in size. One advantage of this is an increased depth of focus. Similar to decreasing the aperture of a camera, when the pupil is very small, the depth of the image being viewed is increased. A small pupil increases the range that an object can be moved back and forth and still kept in focus.

Normal Perceptual Changes of the Aging Eye

Along with physical changes in the aging eye, perceptual changes in the visual system also occur. The accuracy and speed of interpreting visual information decreases with age. For example, visual acuity as it pertains to reading the eye chart, decreases in the older individual. A person who had 20/15 vision when he was 18 probably will only see 20/20 or 20/25 at age 70. The vision is still good but not as sharp as it was 50 years before.

The older individual will not be as sensitive to small changes in his eyeglass prescription as when he was younger. His visual system will not be as discerning. For example, prescriptions are measured in optical units call diopters in increments of 0.25. A young individual can notice prescription changes of 0.25 quite easily. An older individual, on the other hand, will usually not be as sensitive to small changes.

Older individuals also find it more difficult reading print that is not very dark or print that is crowded together. The latter is called the "crowding effect." Neighboring words seem to interfere with the recognition of the word being viewed. The crowding effect can occur in younger individuals as well. However, combined with other aging changes, the "crowding effect" further hinders visual perception in older people.

With aging, there is also a reduction in contrast sensitivity. Contrast sensitivity testing measures the amount of contrast a person needs to see targets of various sizes. Older adults need more of a contrast between small objects and their background in order to view the object clearly. There is a reduction in contrast sensitivity and it makes objects appear washed out. The reduced perception of contrast is probably due to neural changes in the visual pathway.

Another concern is dynamic visual acuity. Reading an eye chart is a measurement of static visual acuity; the viewing object does not move. A more useful measurement of acuity is dynamic visual acuity where the acuity of a moving target is measured. This is more similar to the real world where objects are continually moving. A person will use dynamic visual acuity when driving and trying to spot an exit.

The Eye and Aging: Sub-normal Vision

With the advancing years, there is a reduction in dynamic visual acuity probably greater than the reduction in static visual acuity. The sensitivity for recognizing moving objects simply decreases.

Aging also affects peripheral vision. The peripheral or side vision is not as sharp, possibly because of a reduced retinal metabolism. The visual field of an older individual also shrinks.

The constriction of the visual field can hamper driving and other mobility tasks. When an object enters the visual field from the periphery, the older adult's reaction time will be increased. The recognition of the object will take longer. This can, obviously, affect driving.

Another aspect of visual perception is dark adaptation. Dark adaptation is the process of attaining visual comfort when leaving a bright environment and entering a dark room. The classic example is entering a movie theater on a sunny day. The eyes will take a few minutes to adapt to the dark environment.

In the bright sunlight, the cones in the retina are functioning primarily. When entering the dark movie theater, the cones reduce their function and the rods must be stimulated. The rods are responsible for vision in dim illumination. This process of converting form a photopic (cone stimulated) to a scotopic (rod stimulated) system takes a few minutes and is called dark adaptation.

Older adults take longer adapting to a dark environment after being exposed to a bright light. They may bump into objects after entering a dimly lit room. Clinically, dark adaptation can be measured by how fast a person responds to a bright test target after entering a dark room. People with poor dark adaptation will respond either very slowly to the test target or will require a much brighter test target than normal.

Generally speaking, if the older adult has healthy eyes, the reduction in dark adaptation is not a serious problem.

Glare, however, is a very real problem for the older adult. Because of the normal aging changes of the lens, incoming light is scattered within the eye creating glare. Glare reduces the sensitivity to a viewed object.

Glare when driving at night is particularly troublesome. The headlights form oncoming cars can literally blind the driver. This type of glare is called disability glare and it is annoying to everyone, more so with senior citizens, however.

YOUR EYES!

When facing oncoming headlights, some drivers find it necessary to temporarily close the left eye or simply direct their gaze to the right until the car
passes. Anti-reflective coatings on eyeglasses can sometimes help.

Visual performance in an unfamiliar environment can also be compromised
with aging vision. Older individuals tend to react slowly when localizing objects in their visual field. Insignificant objects can become distracting. For
example, when driving and attempting to identify a sign, other signs, headlights and buildings interfere with the identification process. This localization
of an object becomes more trying with advancing age.

Observing details obscured by shadows also becomes more difficult. Driving in bright sunlight down a road lined with trees creates a high contrast situation. The driver must constantly adjust his vision from areas of brightness
to areas of shadows (when the trees block the sun). Rapidly switching back
and forth from dim illumination to bright illumination tends to become more
difficult with age.

The high illumination areas, where the sunlight penetrates freely, act as a
distracting background and make viewing details in the shaded areas harder
to detect. With the aging eye, the processing of stimuli in the shaded areas
becomes slower. In other words, the reaction time is longer.

Many senior citizens find driving during the twilight hours harder than when
they were younger. The reduced illumination causes a problem in identifying
details. Viewing during twilight is transitional; not the bright illuminance of
daytime and not quite the dark adaptation of night time. Many people find
this annoying.

Finally, the aging eye can have difficulty identifying certain colors, most notably shades of blue. As was mentioned earlier, the lens of the eye takes on a
yellowish brown appearance as it ages. The yellow in the aging lens absorbs
incoming blue light before it can reach the retina. The more yellow the aging
lens, the more the color blue is filtered out; and hence, the more difficult is the
perception of the color blue. The same effect can be noticed by wearing yellow sunglasses. Shades of blue will be more difficult to perceive.

In order to perceive colors as they actually are, older individuals need bright
illumination. The brighter the light, the truer the colors will appear. Dim illumination, such as twilight viewing, can cause much difficulty with color
perception.

Overall, visual perception in the older adult is not as quick and as accurate as
it was in youth. Most of the changes are slow developing and have only a

minor impact on vision. It is important to realize that these changes are normal aging changes which develop in all eyes to some degree. An abnormal or a diseased state would involve the speeding up or the exaggeration of these conditions.

Subnormal Vision: Visual Devices for the Impaired

Subnormal vision (visual impairment) does not result from normal aging changes but rather from disease processes. The four major diseases of the elderly population which can lead to visual impairment are: glaucoma, macular degeneration, diabetic retina disease and cataracts.

Subnormal vision is also called low vision. Low vision is abnormal visual acuity or reduced visual fields because of a disorder of the visual system. The defect can be anywhere in the visual system: the eye, the visual pathway or the visual cortex in the brain. The condition can be congenital or acquired later in life.

The disease process leads to irreversible, bilateral subnormal vision. Medicine, surgery and standard optical devices, such as eyeglasses and contacts, cannot improve vision to normal levels.

Visual acuity can be within normal limits, but the visual field can be severely impaired. For a visual field problem to be considered an impairment, it must restrict normal performance.

Definitions

Legal Blindness

Legal blindness is best corrected visual acuity of 20/200 or less in the better seeing eye or a central field of 20 degrees or less. This means that conventional lenses (eyeglasses or contacts) cannot improve vision better than 20/200. Visual acuity can be within normal limits but a person with a visual field of 20 degrees or less in the horizontal direction is considered legally blind.

Low Vision

The definition of low vision is best corrected visual acuity of 20/70 or less in the better seeing eye or a central field of 30 degrees or less in the horizontal direction.

YOUR EYES!

Functionally Blind

A functionally blind individual may be able to perceive form perception or light perception but has very little usable vision. The person functions as a blind individual.

Totally Blind

A totally blind individual has no ability to detect light in either eye. This condition is rare; most blind individuals can detect either form or light to some degree.

Disability

A disability means that the individual is unable to perform a particular task. A person can have a visual impairment but have no difficulty performing normal activities. This individual would not be considered disabled.

Visual Impairment

Visual impairment can affect performance in a variety of ways. Reduced visual acuity results from loss of macular function. The macula is responsible for the sharpest vision.

An abnormal visual field can either be from a loss of macular function (a central field defect) or from a peripheral retinal disorder such as constricted fields.

Night blindness results from a disorder of the rods which are responsible for vision in dim illumination. This person will have no problem during the day but will have great difficulty seeing in faint illumination. An abnormal dark adaptation implies that the rods are not sufficiently stimulated when going from bright illumination to dim illumination.

Some disorders, such as strabismus, prevent fusion of the images from both eyes. A macular disorder can also prevent image fusion since the central vision is destroyed. Loss of fusion results in the loss of stereoscopic vision and depth perception.

Visual impairment can also affect color vision. The condition can be congenital where a defect of the photoreceptors is present at birth. The condition can also be acquired, such as optic nerve inflammation, where a red color defect may develop.

The Eye and Aging: Sub-normal Vision

When a person has a visual impairment, several steps can be taken to improve their visual performance. The most obvious is trying conventional lenses (eyeglasses or contacts). If conventional lenses cannot improve vision, low vision optical devices can be tried. The magnifying aids can be designed to improve either distance or near vision.

Very often, the low vision patient must undergo extensive training to learn new viewing techniques. Psychological counseling is often required.

Magnification

Everyone is familiar with magnifying lenses. People use binoculars or hand held magnifying lenses all of the time. Spectators at ballgames use binoculars to watch the action, stamp collectors use a magnifying lens to view small details on the stamps. Telescopes are used to view the stars.

Magnification is the cornerstone of vision rehabilitation with low vision aids. There is a major difference between people with normal vision using magnifying aids and people with subnormal vision using them. Individuals with subnormal vision **need** the aids in order to perform their visual activities. People with normal vision use the visual devices for a particular task but can perform their normal daily activities without the use of magnifying devices.

For individuals with normal vision, magnification is a luxury. For people with subnormal vision, magnification is a necessity if they wish to function visually.

People with normal vision sometimes have difficulty understanding the trauma involved with vision rehabilitation. They can see fine with or without visual aids. The low vision patient, on the other hand, needs the magnification devices in order to keep in touch with the visual aspects of the real world. Without magnification, he is lost.

Magnification can be achieved in different ways. Simply by enlarging the viewing object, linear magnification can be produced. Large, bold print in newspapers and magazines are examples of linear magnification. Many low vision patients do well with large print books. When writing a letter or signing a check, broad tipped pens can be used to produce bolder and more visible print.

Another type of magnification is relative distance magnification. This is accomplished by bringing the viewing material closer to the eye. The closer the material is to the eye, the larger the image appears on the retina. Relative distance magnification is used frequently by low vision patients for both distance and near objects.

The third type of magnification is angular magnification. This is the type produced by a lens system, either a telescope or a microscope. A telescope will make distant objects appear closer and a microscope will make print appear closer to the eye. In low vision terminology, very strong magnifying spectacles are called microscopes.

Telescopes and microscopes are optical aids. They are used to enhance the visual performance of low vision patients. The optical devices divert incoming light rays away from diseased retinal tissue onto healthy tissue to maximize visual awareness.

The optical aids generally serve a specific function and various devices may be prescribed for different tasks. No one device is ideally suited for all visual demands. The optical devices are prescribed based on the type and severity of the visual condition and the patient's responses to the devices.

The Low Vision Evaluation

The low vision evaluation, particularly the initial examination, is long and often trying for the patient. Much information must be gathered by the low vision specialist. A low vision specialist is almost always an optometrist who has had extensive training in evaluating subnormal vision and fitting and analyzing low vision devices.

An important consideration during the initial evaluation is the length of time the vision has been impaired. If the vision loss is recent, patients usually are not receptive to visual aids. An adjustment period is required for the anger and bitterness to subside. The patient often seeks further medical help in the hope that lost vision can be restored. After all medical and surgical possibilities have been exhausted, the patient may then be receptive to optical aids.

A person who has accepted his visual condition is more likely to be motivated enough to attempt vision rehabilitation through the use of optical aids. During the evaluation, the vision specialist will pay careful attention to the emotional state of the patient.

The patient's health history is extremely important. All eye diseases, previous treatments and medications are noted. The patient is asked if he understands his condition and the visual restrictions it has imposed on him. The patient must understand why visual devices are necessary before he will accept them.

Each eye disorder affects visual function differently. The low vision specialist must determine exactly how the visual disorder is reducing visual function before he can prescribe the appropriate optical aids. The optometrist will carefully measure best corrected distance and near visual acuities. This will be important for later calculations. The patient's visual fields will also be determined. A full eye health evaluation will also be performed.

The stability of the eye disorder is also an important consideration. If the condition is likely to deteriorate in time, the prognosis for vision rehabilitation is guarded. If the condition is stable, the optical devices can be prescribed with much more confidence.

The family history is also important. If the vision loss is from a genetic disorder, other family members need to be examined. Genetic counseling may also be recommended.

The patient's mobility will also be assessed. Mobility refers to how well the patient moves about inside or outside his home. Many individuals with subnormal vision are afraid to venture outdoors in an unfamiliar environment. Sometimes, they have difficulty avoiding obstacles in their own home.

The patient will be asked if he has any difficulty moving about the house or has any problems with traveling. These issues must be addressed during the evaluation.

Lighting can also be a problem for the low vision patient. The patient's home lighting is a consideration when prescribing magnifying devices. Generally speaking, the brighter the light, the more the vision is enhanced with the use of magnification. Special lamps or brighter light bulbs are often recommended.

Outdoor lighting and glare can also be a problem. A person with a retinal disorder affecting the rods will have no problem with daytime vision but night vision will be drastically reduced. A person with macular disease, on the other hand, will have most of his visual difficulties during the daytime. Sunlight and glare will make daytime mobility practically impossible.

Questions will be asked of the low vision patient concerning his hobbies and activities. Specific tasks require specific visual aids. The complexity and working distance of the activity must also be considered. A patient wishing to view street signs will do well with a hand held telescope. A patient wishing to play the piano, on the other hand, will probably need some type of spectacle mounted microscope or telescope.

The prescribing of low vision aids must be task oriented. Low vision patients who wish to perform a specific task or achieve a specific goal do much better with visual aids than patients who simply "want to see better."

Patients who simply want to see better often have unrealistic expectations. Optical devices cannot substitute for the healthy human eye. They can permit the properly motivated low vision patient some freedom from his visual restrictions, however.

Low vision devices, particularly telescopes, are quite expensive and require much time and effort on the part of both the doctor and the patient. But for low vision patients who cannot achieve functional vision by any other means, optical devices with vision rehabilitation can make a remarkable difference.

Loss of Functional Vision from Disease

Basically, there are three major types of functional vision loss: overall blurred vision without a field loss, a central field defect or a peripheral field defect. The peripheral defect can either be a constricted field (no side vision) or a hemianopic defect. With a right hemianopia, for example, the right half of each eye has no vision.

Any abnormalities of the refractive structures of the eye (the media) can cause overall blurred vision. Any disorder affecting the cornea, lens or vitreous can inhibit light transmission to the retina. The reduced light retards the visual image and results in blurred vision. There is no field defect present. The entire visual field is intact but the whole field is blurred. *(Figure 10-1)*

Problems with the cornea include congenital degenerations of corneal tissue, edema and corneal scarring. Lens disorders are, obviously, cataracts. Vitreal clouding usually results from dead cells from an infection or blood leaking into the vitreous from a retinal hemorrhage.

All of these conditions result in similar symptoms, primarily reduced visual acuity. The patient experiences hazy vision because of the disruption of the normally clear media.

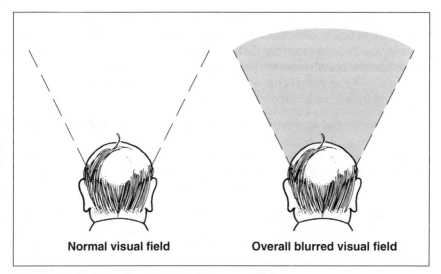

Normal visual field   Overall blurred visual field

Figure 10-1   The visual field with overall blur.

Glare is another major problem when the media is clouded. It is more pronounced in bright sunlight since there is more incoming light to be distorted and scattered.

When overall blurred vision is the problem, controlling illumination is the most important consideration. Any device that filters incoming light is useful. Tints and ultraviolet filters are frequently used as well as anti-reflective coatings. Sunglasses with tinted side shields also increase visual comfort. Gray filters are often used for cataract patients and yellow filters help improve contrast for patients with corneal opacities.

Special tinted absorptive lenses, by Corning, have been very successful in eliminating glare, poor vision and light sensitivity. The Corning lenses are photochromatic; they become darker in bright illumination and the tint becomes less dark in dimmer light.

There are three shades of the Corning lens: CPF 550 (red), CPF 527 (orange) and CPF 511 (yellow). The lenses increase contrast while minimally distorting color perception. (Colored lenses do block light, however. A colored lens primarily blocks its opposite color. A red lens, for example, blocks green light and a yellow lens blocks blue light).

Patients who are sensitive to fluorescent lights or who have mobility problems because of curbs or steps do very well with all the Corning lenses. The

Corning lenses are somewhat expensive but the reduction in glare and improvement in acuity and contrast can be remarkable. The lenses can improve vision for everyone, not just low vision patients. However, they are used primarily for patients with hazy vision due to media opacities, such as cataracts. These conditions would result in scattering of incoming light causing glare and reduced contrast.

The second type of functional vision loss is a central field defect. *(Figure 10-2)* Any defect in the macula or the retinal tissue immediately surrounding the macula, in an area of thirty degrees or less, involves the central field. The cones are predominantly situated in this area. Damage to the cones can result in a loss of color vision as well as a loss of acuity.

Many visual disorders can cause a central field defect. Optic nerve disease as well as certain toxic substances such as methyl alcohol or lead can wipe out the central vision. Trauma to the back of the eye or a hole in the macula can also cause a central defect.

Macular disease is the most common cause of a central field defect, in particular, senile macular degeneration.

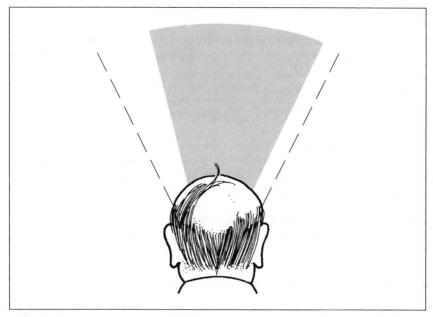

Figure 10-2 Central field defect.

A central field defect is often reported by patients as a distortion, an area of blurred vision or simply "not there." It does not appear as a large black spot in the center of the patient's vision. Very often, the patient will not be able to read and will have difficulty seeing fine details. They will also not be able to see a person's face at a distance.

A major clue to a central field defect is when the patient says that they can see better when looking slightly off center. The patient is directing his gaze to an area of healthy retinal tissue adjacent to the diseased area. Since he is not looking with his macula, the vision will not be particularly sharp. It will be more comfortable then when looking through the defect, however.

Another clue to a central field defect is the inability to detect the color red. In mild cases of macular or optic nerve disease, the perception of the color red is diminished.

Patients with central field defects can often successfully substitute their side vision in place of their central vision. The defect only occupies a fraction of the visual field. Because of this, low vision patients with a central field defect react favorably to visual aids. Magnification works particularly well.

Moving objects closer to the eye (relative distance magnification) works nicely. It increases the size of the retinal image while decreasing the portion of the total image where the defect is located.

Magnification devices, such as telescopes or very strong reading corrections (microscopes), improve vision by spreading the optical image onto healthy retinal tissue. The amount of magnification needed depends on the extent of the visual field defect and the visual requirements of the patient.

A magnification device in the form of glasses usually gives better results than hand held magnifiers. It is difficult to align the eyes with a hand held magnifier and it requires additional coordination.

The greater the magnification, the closer the viewing object must be held to the eye. For comfortable viewing, the viewing object cannot be moved abruptly.

Microscopic eyeglasses are probably the best optical device for the patient with a central field defect. Learning to read with the lenses requires much patience and training. Any slight head movement causes the viewing area to move excessively and can be frustrating in the beginning. The normal method of moving the eyes across the page when reading causes problems because the movement is magnified. Sometimes, it is easier if the patient holds his head still and moves the reading material from right to left while reading from left to right. This, obviously, requires practice.

The final type of functional vision loss is a peripheral field defect. *(Figure 10-3)* This type of defect is usually more disabling than a central defect or overall blurred vision.

A constricting type of visual field defect can result from glaucoma or a peripheral retinal disease such as retinitis pigmentosa. The end result of a constricting field defect would be the destruction of all vision except for a small area in the central field. It would have the same effect as someone with normal vision looking through a straw all day. Obviously, mobility would be a major problem.

The other type of peripheral field defect is a hemianopia: the vision of the right or left half of both eyes is wiped out. This can develop after a stroke; the oxygen supply to a side of the brain is cut off resulting in a visual field defect on the opposite side.

A person with a constricted visual field gets less information the closer the object is to his eye. Bringing reading material closer makes viewing more

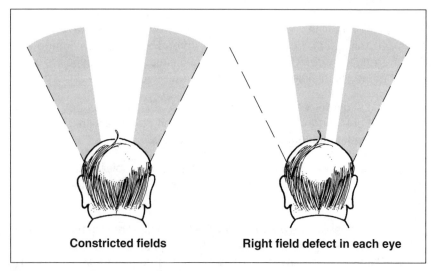

Constricted fields   **Right field defect in each eye**

Figure 10-3   Peripheral field defects.

difficult. Magnification does not work well with peripheral field defects since the enlarged image will be projected into the defective area of the retina.

The peripheral areas of the retina (primarily rods) are responsible for viewing in dim illumination and are also motion detectors. If these areas are destroyed, a person's mobility will be severely restricted. The individual with a peripheral field cut will not be aware of objects approaching him from the sides.

This individual will constantly bump into things and is always looking down at his feet when walking. He becomes very nervous in unfamiliar surroundings. He usually walks with an arm extended outward to protect himself from unseen obstacles.

The individual with a hemianopic field cut will turn his head to the direction of the field defect. If a person has a right hemianopic field loss, he will turn his head to the right allowing easier viewing with his left field which has no defect. This person will be constantly bumping into things on his blind side. If he has a right side defect, he may also have difficulty reading since we read from left to right.

Magnification does not work for peripheral field defects since it further reduces the visual field. Reverse telescopes, also called field expanders, are used for these types of defects. Instead of magnifying the image, they minify it or shrink it. More information is compressed into the residual field.

The problem with reverse telescopes is that by shrinking the image, it reduces visual acuity and causes distortion. Everything looks smaller, but the field is increased. Reverse telescopes are good for spotting tasks but they are not ideal for long term viewing. Walking while wearing a reverse telescope is difficult and uncomfortable.

Low Vision Devices

Microscopes

Magnifying Spectacles

Very strong convex (plus) lenses mounted in eyeglasses are called microscopes. They magnify small print and other close material. Microscopes can be either monocular (mounted over one eye) or binocular (mounted over both eyes).

With microscopes, the image on the retina is enlarged allowing better acuity. The working distance of the lens is fixed; reading material cannot be held any further then the focal distance of the lens.

Spectacle-mounted microscopes are usually offered first to the patient. They are the most acceptable type of visual aid for prolonged reading since the hands are free. Patients who previously had standard reading glasses adapt very easily to these devices. As a rule, the device is mounted monocularly.

Advantages of Spectacle Mounted Lenses:

- psychologically acceptable
- both hands are free
- useful for prolonged reading
- can be monocular or binocular

Disadvantages of Spectacle Mounted Lenses:

- requires very close reading distance
- fixed reading distance, determined by lens power
- reduced reading speed, particularly with the higher powers

Hand Held Magnifiers

Hand held magnifiers are convex lenses mounted with a handle. They are held between the eye and the viewing material. The further the magnifier is from the eye, the smaller the field of view. The magnification is increased as the magnifier is moved closer to the eye.

Advantages of Hand Held Magnifiers:

- can be used while wearing standard glasses
- useful for short term tasks, such as reading labels
- greater working range
- adaptation is easy

Disadvantages of Hand Held Magnifiers:

- reading speed is reduced
- difficult to use if the patient has a hand tremor

- reduced field of view compared to spectacles
- must be held at the correct focal distance

Stand Magnifiers

A stand magnifier is a convex lens mounted in a rigid structure which can be rested over the top of the reading material.

They are used when patients cannot hold a hand magnifier or cannot tolerate the very close working distance of spectacle mounted lenses.

Advantages of Stand Magnifiers:

- normal reading distance
- useful when a patient has constricted fields
- useful for short term tasks
- predictable fixed focal length

Disadvantages of Stand Magnifiers:

- reduced visual field
- leaning over reading material can be uncomfortable
- patient must look directly down into the lens to avoid any peripheral distortion

Telescopes

Distance Telescopes

A telescope is an optical device that improves the clarity of distant objects by enlarging their image size. They bring the object closer through the use of angular magnification. A telescope consists of two lenses placed together at a fixed distance. The lens closest to the eye is called the ocular and the lens furthest from the eye is called the objective.

There are two types of telescopes: Galilean and Keplerian. The more simple of the two is the Galilean telescope. The ocular lens is concave (minus) and the objective lens is convex (plus). This produces an upright image when the lenses are separated by their focal length.

A more sophisticated telescope is the Keplerian. In a Keplerian system, both the ocular and the objective lenses are convex. This results in an inverted image. The image is made erect by the use of internal prisms.

YOUR EYES!

The optics of a Keplerian telescope are far superior to the optics of a Galilean telescope. The field of view is also larger and the light transmission is better with a Keplerian system.

The field of view through a telescope is limited by the diameter of the objective lens. With all telescopes, the field of view is widest when the telescope is held as close to the eye as possible.

Telescopes can be either monocular or binocular, hand held or mounted in a spectacle frame. They usually have an adjustable focus. Telescopes are generally much more difficult for the doctor to fit and the patient to adapt to compared to microscopic systems.

Advantages of Telescopes for Distance:

- only system that can provide distance magnification
- can be used for traveling and spotting tasks

Disadvantages of Telescopes for distance:

- extra training is required
- reduced field of view
- difficulty finding objects and focusing
- expensive

Near Telescopes

A near telescope is an adjustable focus telescope mounted for near viewing in a spectacle frame. They are prescribed for patients who want an extended working distance for near tasks.

Advantages of Near Telescopes:

- adjustable working distance
- both hands are free
- can be focused for intermediate range tasks such as reading or working at a computer screen

Disadvantages of Near Telescopes:

- depth of field is very critical; slight head movements distort the image
- the field of view is smaller than a spectacle mounted convex lens (a microscope)

Closed Circuit Television for Reading

A closed circuit television reading device is a television camera which relays a magnified image to a monitor. The patient can sit at a normal reading distance. The magnified reading material is displayed on the television screen. The magnification is controlled by a zoom lens which is adjustable.

The magnification can be varied at will and the normal reading distance is less tiring than other optical devices. It is ideal for students and professionals who are visually impaired and must do a lot of reading.

Advantages of Closed Circuit Television for Reading:

- greater range of magnification as opposed to spectacles
- can be used binocularly
- can be used for writing and typing
- normal reading distance

Disadvantages of Closed Circuit Television for Reading:

- units are very expensive
- units are bulky
- reading speed may be too slow for some patients

Sources for Eye Information

American Foundation for the Blind
15 West 16th Street
New York, NY, 10011
212-620-2170

American Diabetes Association
600 Fifth Avenue
New York, NY, 10017
212-541-4310

National Association for the Visually Handicapped
305 East 24th Street
New York, NY, 10010
212-889-3141

National Eye Institute
Information Offices
Building 31 – Room 6125
Bethesda, MD, 20205
301-496-5248

The National Retinitis Pigmentosa Foundation
8331 Mindale Circle
Baltimore, MD, 21207
301-655-1011

11

Closing Thoughts

The Need for Prevention

"An ounce of prevention is worth a pound of cure" is certainly true for eye-care. In many cases where prevention is possible, it is much better to take precautions than to rely on treatment after the condition is established.

A classic case for eyecare prevention is the condition called retrolental fibro-plasia (RLF). Retrolental fibroplasia is a potentially blinding disease that af-fects premature infants. Research has shown that high oxygen levels ad-ministered to premature infants can contribute to the disease. The artificially high oxygen levels can cause changes in the retinal blood vessels leading to unnatural vessel growth and eventual blindness.

The oxygen levels are regulated much more carefully nowadays. The treat-ment for retrolental fibroplasia is not particularly successful; the key to re-ducing the incidence of blindness in newborns is prevention.

Another example of prevention in eyecare is the treatment for amblyopia or "lazy eye." With amblyopia, the eye becomes weak from lack of use.

YOUR EYES!

Occluding the good eye, forcing the weaker eye to work, prevents irreversible damage to binocular function. Amblyopia therapy is performed aggressively at an early age to prevent the loss of vision from becoming established. After many years of poor vision, an amblyopic eye responds very poorly to treatment.

Correcting refractive disorders, vision therapy and other treatments at an early age allow the child to be at his best visually. This encourages proper development during the early learning years. Parents should be wary of a child who covers one eye, rubs his eyes excessively, tilts his head or gets very close to objects.

Most eye injuries in the working environment, at home and in sports can be prevented. The key is proper use of eye safety equipment. Parents should also check their children's toys for sharp edges and educate them about eye safety.

The development of cataracts, although related to aging, can be slowed appreciably by limiting exposure to ultraviolet light. Proper eye protection when outdoors will prevent unnecessary ultraviolet light exposure and reduce the aging process of the lens of the eye.

The development of macular degeneration, again related to aging, can also be lessened somewhat by limiting the exposure of the retina to ultraviolet light. The more pale an individual's complexion is, the more susceptible he is to macular degeneration. Again, protective eyewear with an ultraviolet filter is in order. When macular degeneration becomes established, there is no cure.

Diabetes is another condition where controlling the disorder in the early stages may prevent further complications. It is imperative that the diabetic patient maintains reasonably stable blood sugar levels throughout life. Regular medical and dilated eye health evaluations are mandatory.

As with any condition, the earlier the treatment, the better the chance for success. Diabetes and its many complications should not be taken lightly.

The prevention of glaucoma requires regular eye examinations for the measurement of the intraocluar pressure and an assessment of the optic nerve and visual field. Glaucoma presents with no obvious symptoms.

Untreated glaucoma for an extended period of time will cause irreversible vision loss and possibly total blindness. Early detection and subsequent treatment is the key.

The prevention of contact lens problems simply requires following the instructions for the proper care and handling of the lenses. Only the recommended solutions should be used. At the first sign of a serious problem: pain, redness, very blurry vision, the contacts should be removed and the patient should seek help immediately.

The prevention of visually related problems of elderly patients, particularly when driving, bears mentioning. Because of reduced visual function, elderly drivers must take precautions.

Senior citizens who drive should avoid driving at night or twilight. They should also wear sunglasses for daytime driving. In addition, they should keep their eyeglasses and windshields clean since dirty glass can contribute to glare and also reduce vision.

When driving, they should try to get the overall picture and check their rear-view mirror frequently. Finally, they should attempt to use their peripheral vision more instead of directing their vision constantly straight ahead.

An individual's vision and eye health are related to his overall health and well-being. The eyes are not isolated from the rest of the body; a person's lifestyle, diet and health can all affect the eyes.

The following will not only benefit the eyes but, obviously, the entire body and well being of the individual:

- proper nutrition: limiting fats and salt and increasing dietary fiber. Multiple vitamin supplements with ample supplies of Vitamin A, Vitamin C and vitamin E for the eyes. Drink plenty of water.

- regular exercise, stressing aerobics

- limiting alcoholic intake and other drugs

- reducing stress

- not smoking

- maintaining a normal body weight

- using proper eye protection, including an ultraviolet filter

- having regular medical, dental and eye examinations

Sources for Eye Information

Dictionary of Eye Terminology
by Barbara Cassin
Gainsville, Florida. Triad, 1984

Dictionary of Visual Science
by David Cline
Radnor, Pennsylvania. Chilton Books, 1980

NSPB Information Center
79 Madison Avenue
New York, NY 10016
212-684-3505

NSPB has over 3,000 volumes on eye health, safety, optometry, ophthalmology, medicine, public health and prevention of blindness. They will provide information on eyecare. If they cannot provide the information requested, they will refer to the appropriate source.

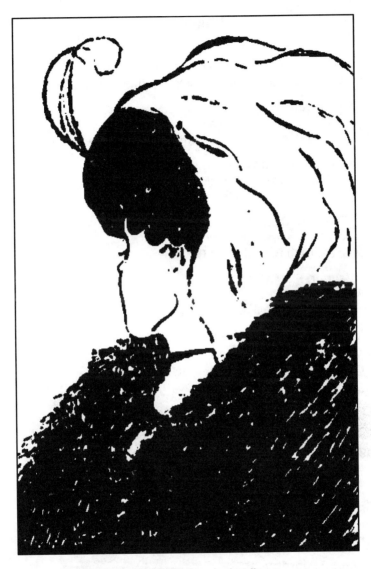

Figure 11-1 "My Wife and My Mother-in-law"
An ambiguous figure which can be viewed in two ways.
It may be perceived as either a "mother-in-law" or the left
profile of a young woman. (from E. G. Boring, American
Journal of Psychology, vol 42, 1930)

Bibliography

Barnhart, Edward, R.
Physician's Desk Reference of Ophthalmology.
Oradell: Medical Economics Company, Inc., 1989.

Barnhart, Edward, R.
Physician's Desk Reference.
Oradell: Medical Economics Company, Inc., 1989.

Bartlett, D. Jimmy and Jaanus, siret, D.
Clinical Ocular Pharmacology.
Boston: Butterworth, 1984.

Duane, Thomas, D., M.D.
Clinical Ophthalmology Volumes I thru V.
Philadelphia: J.B. Lippincott C., 1989.

Faye, Eleanor, E., M.D.
Clinical Low Vision.
Boston: Little, Brown and Co., 1984.

Friel, John, P.
Dorland's Medical Dictionary.
Philadelphia: W.B. Saunders Company, 1981.

Gray, Henry, F.R.S.
Gray's Anatomy.
New York: Bounty Books, 1977.

Gregg, James, R.
Vision and Sports.
Boston: Butterworth, 1987.

Griffin, John, R., O.D.
Binocular Anomalies: Procedures for Vision Therapy.
Chicago: Professional Press, Inc., 1982.

Grosvenor, Theordore, P.
Primary Care Optometry: A Clinical Manual.
Chicago: The Professional Press, 1982.

Haessler, F. Herbert, M.D.
Eye Signs in General Disease.
Springfield: Thomas Books, 1960.

Hurtt, Jane, R.N., A.A., Rasicovici, Antonia, B.A., Windsor, C. E. M.D.
Comprehensive Review of Orthoptics and Ocular Motility: Theory, Therapy and Surgery.
Saint Louis: C.V. Bosby Co., 1972.

Kanski, Jack, J.
The Eye in Systemic Disease.
Boston: Butterworth, 1986.

Langston, Deborah Pavan, M.D.
Manual of Ocular Diagnosis and Therapy.
Boston: Little, Brown and Company, 1980.

Mandell, Robert, B.
Contact Lens Practice.
Springfield: Charles C. Thomas, 1981.

Newell, Frank W.
Ophthalmology: Principles and Concepts.
St. Louis: C.V. Mosby Company, 1982.

Rodgin, J., O.D.
Pathology and Pharmacology of the Eye.
Chicago: The Professional Press, Inc., 1983.

Rosner, Jerome, O.D.
Pediatric Optometry.
Boston: Butterworth, 1981.

Rubin, Melvin, L.
Optics for Clinicians.
Gainesville: Triad Scientific Publishers, 1977.

Vaughn, Daniel, M.D. and Asbury Taylor, M.D.
General Ophthalmology.
Los Altos: Lange Medical Publications, 1983.

List of Figures

List of Figures (con't)

A

abducens nerve, 30
acanthamoeba infection, 83
accommodation, 21
accommodative and convergence
systems, 10
accommodative disorders, 100
accommodative dysfunctions, 131
accommodative excess, 100
accommodative infacility (ill-
sustained accommodation),
101
accommodative insufficiency, 100
accommodative system, 111
adie's syndrome, 23
adult-onset diabetes, 166
afferent system, 49
"after cataract",194
afterimage, 45
age-related macular disease, 162
aging cornea, 210
aging eye, 210
aging retina, 210
AIDS, 169
albinism, 172
alcohol, 173
allergic, 151
amaurosis fugax, 169
amber tints, 138
amblyopia, 60, 102, 231
amblyopia (functional), 102
amblyopia ex anopsia, 103
aneurysm, 28, 107
anisometropia, 62
anisometropic amblyopia, 103
anti-reflective coating, 69, 221
antibiotics, 149, 193, 199, 201
aperture rule, 113

aphakia, 90
aqueous fluid, 32
argon laser, 195
arteriolsclerosis, 169
artificial tears, 84, 148, 186
astigmatism, 59, 86
auditory visual integration, 118
automated peripheral field
computer, 130
awareness, 56

B

bacterial infection, 150
bifocal, 61
bifocal types and other
multifocals, 67
bilateral integration, 118
binocular anomalies, 99
binocular function, 232
binocular system, 111
binocular vision and stereopsis, 47
binocularity, 106
blepharitis, 148
blepharoplasty, 197
blink rate, 17
blink reflex, 15
blinking techniques, 77
blood pressure, 13
blowout fracture of the orbit, 21, 145
blue arcs of the retina, 49
brain, 25, 33, 42
brightness sensitivity, 47
brock string, 112
bruch's membrane, 33
bulging eye, 174
Butterfield, George, 73

C

cardiovascular disease, 168

optic nerve, 28, 159
optic radiations, 25
optic tracts, 25
optical aids, 218
optician, 1, 4
optics, 35
optometrist, 1
orbicularis oculi muscle, 17
orbit, 20
orbital cellulitis, 21
OSHA, 140
over-the-counter-medications, 186
overall blurred vision, 220
oxygen, 74, 84, 231

P

panretinal photocoagulation, 205
parallel, 35
paralytic, 107
patches, 108
patient history, 4
pediatric eyecare, 3
pediatric opthalmologist, 107
pediatric optometrist, 107
pediatric optometry, 3
perceptual deficiencies, 118
peripheral vision, 56, 130, 213
peripheral field defect, 224
peripheral retinal disorder, 216
photochromatic lenses, 66, 71, 221
photopic response, 43
photoreceptors, 163
pinhole camera, 37
plastic, 66, 73
plus lenses, 57, 97, 99, 101
polarization, 138
polarizing lenses, 72

polycarbonate, 66, 138
polymethylmethacrylate (PMMA), 74
posterior vitreous detachments, 32
presbyopia, 61, 101, 211
preservatives, 189
prevention, 231
primary colors, 44
prism, 37, 62, 109
prism diopters, 40
processing, 33
prodome, 51
progressive, 67
pseudotumor cerebri (false tumor of the brain), 52
ptosis, 28, 148
pupil, 22, 211
pupillary response, 11
pursuits, 129

R

radial keratotomy, 63
radiation, 145
radiation trauma, 144
reading, 61
reduced visual acuity, 220
removing the eye, 206
retina, 32, 35, 162, 182, 196
  retinal artery occlusion, 169
  retinal blood vessels, 167
  retinal detachment, 164
  retinal detachment, 32
  retinal detachment surgery, 196
  retinal hemorrhages, 167
  retinal laser surgery, 204
  retinal pigment changes, 172
  retinal tear, 204
retinitis pigmentosa, 44, 165, 224
retrolental fibroplasia, 231
rhodopsin, 42

rod stimulated, 213
rods, 33
Rohm and Haas, 73
rubella (german measles), 171

S

saccades, 129
saccadic fixator, 129
safety lenses, 66
sarcoidosis, 171
sclera, 30
scleral buckle, 196
scleritis, 31
scotopic response, 43
scratch resistant coating, 69
senile macular degeneration, 163, 206
senior citizens, 185, 233
sickle cell anemia, 205
silicone implants, 196
simultaneous vision, 88
sinuses, 20
sodium fluorescein, 179
solar retinopathy, 166
spatial discrimination, 47
special lenses, 127
speed of recognition, 131
sphincter, 31
sports vision, 3, 127
  athletes, 127
  face shields, 137
  visualization, 131
squint, 62
staph germs, 148
stereopsis, 11
steroid, 175, 193, 197, 198, 201
strabismic amblyopia, 102

strabismus, 62, 104, 172
stroke, 27
stye, 149
sub-normal vision, 209, 215
sun gazing, 165
sunglasses, 221
suppression, 106
surgery on the cornea, 200
surgery on the lacrimal system, 199
systemic drugs, 177

T

taste test, 200
telescopes, 218, 223, 227
  galilean telescope, 227
  keplerian telescope, 228
  near telescope, 228
  reverse telescopes, 225
temporal discrimination, 47
therapy for amblyopia, 116
thimerisol, 189
thyroid disease, 198
tinted absorptive lenses, 138, 221
tinted windshields, 141
toric lenses, 86
totally blind, 216
toxic amblyopia, 103
toxoplasmosis, 170
trabeculectomy, 162, 195
trabecuplasty, 162
transplant, 200
trifocals, 67
trigeminal nerve, 29
trochlear nerve, 29
tropia, 62
tumor, 107

U

ultraviolet coating, 70

TO ORDER ADDITIONAL COPIES OF

YOUR EYES!

Call
1-800-345-0096

Publisher's Distribution Service

$14.95 per book
(includes shipping & handling)

Visa/MasterCard accepted